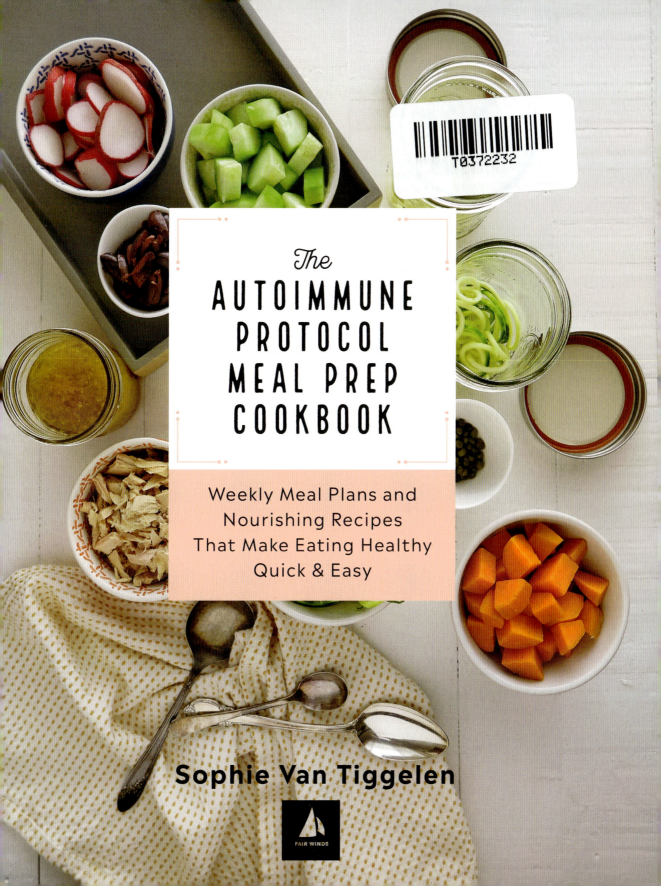

The

AUTOIMMUNE PROTOCOL MEAL PREP COOKBOOK

Weekly Meal Plans and
Nourishing Recipes
That Make Eating Healthy
Quick & Easy

Sophie Van Tiggelen

FAIR WINDS

Quarto.com

© 2020 Quarto Publishing Group USA Inc.
Text © 2020 Sophie Van Tiggelen
Photography © 2020 Quarto Publishing Group USA Inc.

First Published in 2020 by Fair Winds Press, an imprint of The Quarto Group,
100 Cummings Center, Suite 265-D, Beverly, MA 01915, USA.
T (978) 282-9590 F (978) 283-2742

Fair Winds Press titles are also available at discount for retail, wholesale, promotional, and bulk purchase. For details, contact
the Special Sales Manager by email at specialsales@quarto.com or by mail at The Quarto Group, Attn: Special Sales Manager,
100 Cummings Center, Suite 265-D, Beverly, MA 01915, USA.

24   6

ISBN: 978-1-59233-899-3

Digital edition published in 2020
eISBN: 978-1-63159-761-9

Library of Congress Cataloging-in-Publication Data

Tiggelen, Sophie Van, author.
Autoimmune protocol meal prep cookbook : weekly meal plans and
  nourishing recipes that make eating healthy quick & easy / Sophie Van
  Tiggelen.
Beverly, MA : Fair Winds Press, 2019. | Includes index.
ISBN 9781592338993 (trade paperback) | 9781631597619 (eISBN)
1. Autoimmune diseases--Diet therapy--Recipes. 2. Autoimmune
  diseases--Diet therapy. 3. Cookbooks.
LCC RC600 .T542 2019 | DDC 641.5/631--dc23
LCCN 2019025363

Design: Laura Klynstra
Cover Image: Sophie Van Tiggelen
Page Layout: Laura Klynstra
Photography: Sophie Van Tiggelen and photo on page 189 by Lisa Doane Photography (lisadoane.com)

Printed in China

This cookbook is dedicated to

enabling all autoimmune warriors

to cook up a new life

without spending all

your time in the kitchen!

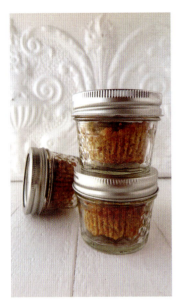
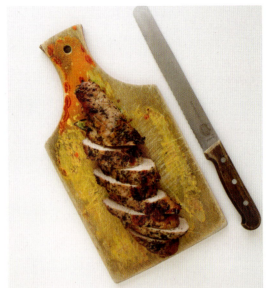
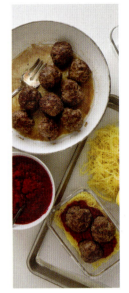
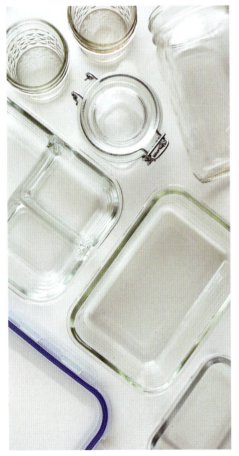
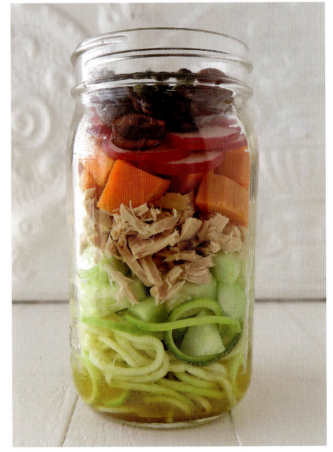

CONTENTS

FOREWORD

Autoimmune disease is an epidemic in our society, affecting an estimated 50 million Americans. Genetics account for about one-third of our risk for autoimmune disease; the rest comes from environmental exposure—like infection, toxins, and pollutants—diet, and lifestyle.

The good news is that immune function is very sensitive to diet and lifestyle choices. By eating well, we support immunoregulatory processes in the body with the net effect of modulating the immune system, decreasing inflammation, and reducing the targeted immune attacks on our tissues that drive autoimmune disease.

The Autoimmune Protocol (AIP) diet is gaining attention as the top health-supportive diet for the millions suffering from autoimmune conditions. Each facet of the diet is supported by scientific evidence, making the AIP a valuable complementary approach to chronic disease management. In a 2017 clinical trial in patients with Inflammatory Bowel Disease, 73 percent of participants were in full clinical remission after following the protocol for only six weeks, and they experienced continued improvement over the entire course of the study. In a 2019 clinical trial on patients with Hashimoto's thyroiditis, patients experienced significant improvement in clinical symptom burden as measured by the Cleveland Clinic Center for Functional Medicine's Medical Symptoms Questionnaire, which decreased from an average of 92 points at the beginning of the study to 29 points after ten weeks of AIP.

However, following AIP tenets does require a sometimes steep learning curve. Many people have no idea where to start or are overwhelmed by the necessary lifestyle shift and diet overhaul, particularly when they are not feeling well.

Whether you are just beginning your AIP journey or are looking to simplify and improve your AIP pathway, *The Autoimmune Protocol Meal Prep Cookbook* is a fantastic resource! You'll get ten weeks of AIP meal plans, including quick and easy recipes, shopping and equipment lists, and batch cooking directions for making all of your meals for the week in one cooking session. Sophie Van Tiggelen makes the AIP accessible so you can jump right into preparing nourishing meals that will support your health. There are numerous meal options including low-FODMAP, low-carb, and one-pot meals, as well as delicious comfort food. Sophie brings her trademark flair to every recipe and her pro tips for storing and reheating will keep every meal delicious.

Health and wellness after an autoimmune diagnosis requires attention to the foods we eat and how we structure our lives, but it doesn't need to be hard or leave us feeling deprived. And with this book at your fingertips, you'll love getting into the kitchen, cooking nourishing AIP meals, and savoring every bite!

–Dr. Sarah Ballantyne, Ph.D.,
New York Times best-selling author of *The Paleo Approach* and *Paleo Principles*

INTRODUCTION

I got really sick in 2009. It happened practically overnight. I started having daily panic attacks, and everything went downhill very quickly from there. Soon I developed severe insomnia—I was sleeping for only two or three hours each night—and was suffering from crippling anxiety. Within the space of a month, I felt like a complete zombie.

I was desperate. I knew something was wrong with me, but my lab tests didn't turn up anything. But what about the swollen thyroid, digestive issues, brain fog, memory loss, heart palpitations, migraines, hair loss, dry skin, muscle weakness, joint pain? I was literally aching for answers. Later that year, I was finally diagnosed with Hashimoto's thyroiditis, an autoimmune disease that attacks the thyroid gland.

Does anything about my story sound familiar to you? If so, take heart. I'm here to show you that full recovery from autoimmune diseases is possible. How did I make this happen? Well, the single most powerful change I made was to rethink the way I ate and to start the Autoimmune Protocol (AIP) diet. Looking back, this simple step has had a profound impact on my recovery. My symptoms improved rapidly and after a year, I felt like my old self again.

Since then, I have spent almost a decade following the AIP to promote healing and to reverse my autoimmune disease. Along the way—through trial and error and lots of experimenting!—I've discovered the best practices for success on AIP. I've figured out what works, what doesn't, and where to invest your time and resources to achieve the best results.

If you have picked up this cookbook, then you already know that the AIP can help you regain your health and feel better. But how can you make this happen in the midst of a busy life—especially when a disease is robbing you of your precious energy?

The answer is: one step at a time, with the help of proven strategies that will allow you to accomplish more with minimal work. That's what this cookbook is all about. When you practice the technique of meal prep to batch-cook your meals, you're sure to have delicious, AIP-compliant meals ready at all times. That way, you can easily keep your diet on track and devote your energy to healing.

Use this book as a powerful tool to help realize your health goals, no matter where you are on your AIP journey. If you're just beginning to implement AIP, the carefully prepared meal plans, shopping lists, and batch-cooking directions in the following pages will smooth your way. And if AIP is already a part of your life, you're sure to love the meal plans for the convenience (and great taste!) they offer.

–Sophie Van Tiggelen

P.S. If you want to learn more about my health journey and the best practices for success with AIP, visit my blog, *A Squirrel in the Kitchen*. www.asquirrelinthekitchen.com

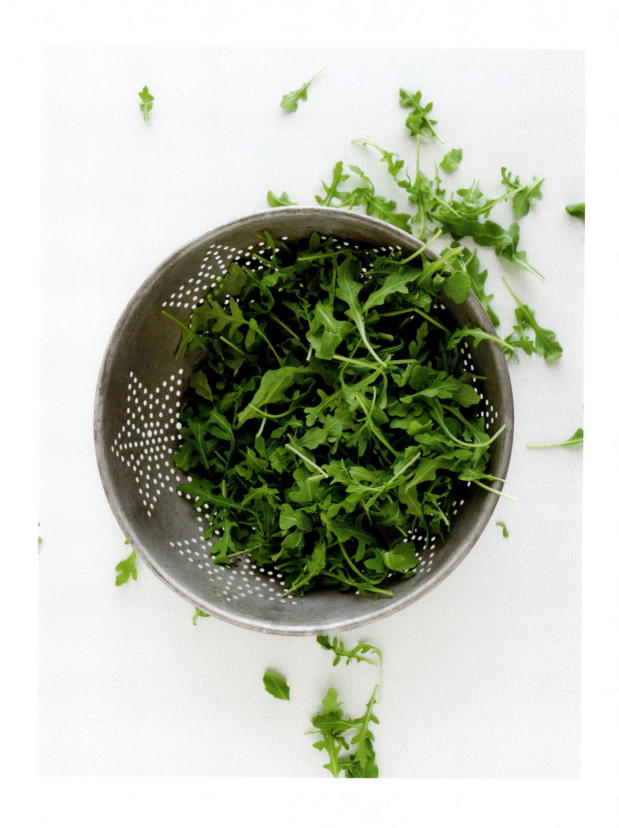

Chapter 1
BENEFITS OF THE AUTOIMMUNE PROTOCOL

What Is the Autoimmune Protocol?

The Autoimmune Protocol, or AIP, is an elimination/reintroduction dietary protocol, focused on nutrient density. It's designed to help determine food intolerances, restore proper immune function, heal the gut, and ultimately eliminate the symptoms of autoimmune disease. The premise is simple: For a limited period of time, you eliminate foods that might trigger intestinal inflammation and stimulate an autoimmune response. This restriction phase is followed by a reintroduction period, during which you gradually reintroduce possible trigger foods to your diet, paying close attention to how your body reacts in order to detect symptoms that may signal a food intolerance.

However, the AIP doesn't work for everyone in exactly the same way. Results vary, depending on how long you've had an autoimmune disease, the severity of your symptoms, and a multitude of other personal and environmental factors, such as the toxins you are exposed to (in personal care products or cleaning supplies, for instance) or your stress levels. For some people, AIP will help alleviate symptoms and provide a better quality of life. Others will be able to achieve complete remission and stop taking their medications. What can it do for you personally? You'll have to give it an honest try to find out!

That said, clinical studies support the effectiveness of AIP. A recent study conducted on the efficacy of the AIP diet for inflammatory bowel disease (more specifically, Crohn's disease and ulcerative colitis) has confirmed what tens of thousands of anecdotal success stories had previously suggested: After six weeks on the AIP, 73 percent of the participants in the study had achieved clinical remission!

Yes, the AIP has been proven to help repair a compromised immune system and restore health. But how is this possible? How can we use food to reverse the cellular damages caused by autoimmune disease? By eliminating harmful, inflammatory foods and replacing them with health-promoting, nutrient-dense ones, AIP targets specific areas known to be instrumental in the emergence and development of autoimmune disease, including the following:

1. **Micronutrient deficiencies.** Your immune system needs vitamins, minerals, antioxidants, essential fatty acids, and amino acids to work correctly.

2. **Inflammation and intestinal permeability.** A healthy microbiome and a healthy gut lining are vital to proper nutrient absorption and optimal immune function.

3. **Blood sugar imbalance.** Sugar highs and lows increase inflammation and trigger autoimmune flares.

4. **Hormonal imbalance.** Your immune system is directly affected by hormonal dysregulation.

By addressing these problem areas and reducing systemic inflammation in the body, AIP helps restore healthy immune function and, over time, can reverse the damage caused by many autoimmune diseases.

How Does the Autoimmune Protocol Work?

Remember that the Autoimmune Protocol is an elimination/reintroduction diet, which means that the initial elimination period isn't meant to last forever. AIP is temporary, so don't worry: Sooner or later you'll get to enjoy a more varied menu again. But until that time, you will focus your energy on removing all the foods that make you sick, while adding a wide variety of nutrient-dense "safe" foods to fuel your recovery.

ELIMINATION

During the elimination period, you should **strictly avoid** grains, gluten, dairy, eggs, legumes (including soy and peanuts), nuts, seeds (including coffee and cocoa), nightshades, alcohol, processed vegetable oils, all food chemicals and additives, and all refined and processed foods. Limit your consumption of high-glycemic-load foods, such as dried fruit, fruit juice, and natural sweeteners like honey and maple syrup. See page 18 for a complete list of ingredients to avoid or eat in moderation.

Instead, **eat plenty of** vegetables and fruit (except nightshades), meat, poultry, organ meat, seafood, fermented foods and drinks (such as sauerkraut and kombucha), bone broth, and healthy fats. See page 17 for a complete list of ingredients to include in your diet.

The elimination period may come as a shock to you. It's easy to focus on all the foods you can't have—but instead, try to switch your attention to all the nourishing foods you still get to enjoy (and, perhaps, all the new foods you're about to discover!). Once you get over the initial hurdle of changing your diet, it can be lots of fun to experiment with new ingredients. View AIP as a culinary adventure—one that will heal you from the inside out.

As you navigate the Autoimmune Protocol, remember to eat as wide a variety of foods as possible from the Foods to Eat list (page 17) and to prioritize locally grown, seasonal products to maximize nutrient diversity. Food quality is also important, but eating organic isn't a requirement when it comes to reaping the benefits of AIP. A cup of conventionally grown broccoli beats an organic doughnut every day of the week!

Throughout the process, it's a good idea to track your symptoms (or the lack of them) in a food journal. This will help you identify any patterns that form.

REINTRODUCTION

After a period of time (and the length of this period is different for each individual), you'll get to reintroduce potential trigger foods into your diet gradually. This will feel really exciting, but it's important not to rush through the reintroduction process, or you risk ruining your results and slowing down your recovery. Remember that the insight you'll gain about your food sensitivities is invaluable for your future health and well-being. So, as a rule of thumb, it's best to wait until all your symptoms have subsided and you have resumed normal life before attempting any reintroduction. For some people, this may take one to three months; for others, it may take over a year. However long it takes for you, try to be patient!

I recommend beginning the reintroduction process on a Saturday morning or another time when you're not working. This will give you plenty of time to make your way through the successive steps without feeling rushed. Here's how to do it:

FOUR-STEP REINTRODUCTION METHOD

Choose **one** food to reintroduce (this is very important: Always reintroduce only one food at a time!).

1. Eat ½ teaspoon of the food and wait 15 minutes. If symptoms appear, stop.

2. Eat 1 teaspoon of the food and wait another 15 minutes. If symptoms appear, stop.

3. Eat 1½ teaspoons and wait 2 to 3 hours. If symptoms appear, stop.

4. Now, eat a normal-size portion and wait 3 to 7 days. Do not reintroduce any other foods during this "waiting" period. If no symptoms appear, you are in the clear.

If symptoms do appear at any time during the reintroduction process, stop consuming the food immediately and wait until the symptoms have completely subsided before giving it another try. If you continue to react to a particular food after several attempts, you may need to avoid this food permanently.

What Can You Expect on the Autoimmune Protocol?

How long will it take for you to start seeing results? When will you feel better? When will your symptoms disappear? When will you regain your energy? There are no universal answers to these questions, and the results you will achieve may range anywhere from a noticeable improvement in your quality of life to full remission of your autoimmune disease.

Your results will be influenced by your genetics, because the "message" contained in your genes can increase your chances of developing one disease or another. Each person has a different genetic "blueprint" that drives everything that happens inside their body, from cholesterol levels to the way they react to stress. Your results will also depend on how long it takes for your gut to heal and your immune system to normalize.

The process of healing from the damage caused by an autoimmune disease takes time and requires patience. After all, it takes years for an autoimmune condition to develop, so it will, in all likelihood, take years to heal! You may read stories online of people turning around

their health and coming off their medications within three months. Such dramatic results aren't impossible, but they are not representative of what the majority of people can expect from AIP.

Still, the important thing to remember is this: Most people report noticeable improvements in their very first month on AIP, with their symptoms gradually receding and even disappearing over time. The healing process resembles a slow and steady journey, not a race to a finish line.

So, the longer you stay on AIP, the more chances you give your gut to heal. It is not at all unusual to be on AIP for as long as a year before your body has recovered enough to be able to handle the reintroduction process.

Your diet is important, but it's not the only factor that influences your recovery. Other aspects affect your recovery, such as:

- Underlying coinfections, such as SIBO (small intestinal bacterial overgrowth), candida, or *H. pylori*

- Hormonal imbalances

- Toxicity due to exposure to environmental factors, such as chemicals in self-care products or heavy metals in food and water

- Lifestyle habits, such as sleep quality, stress management, and exercise

- A tendency to "cheat" on your AIP more than once in a while

A sensitivity to a food that's allowed on the Autoimmune Protocol, which unintentionally keeps your immune system revved up

If you don't see any improvements in your symptoms after three months or you reach a plateau in your healing, talk to your health care practitioner. He or she will be able to order appropriate lab tests and help determine which underlying conditions may be triggering your persistent symptoms.

One final word about managing expectations: There is a difference between remission and a cure. It *is* possible to put your autoimmune disease into remission and live a symptom-free life, and thousands of people have done it thanks to AIP. But remission isn't a cure, and if you start eating the foods that were making you sick before the Autoimmune Protocol, chances are that your symptoms will resurface and your autoimmune condition will be reactivated.

What Makes an AIP Meal?

Now that you are more familiar with how the Autoimmune Protocol works, it's time to get to the fun stuff! Let's take a closer look at what you'll see on your plate in the coming months.

CORE PRINCIPLES

There are a few core principles to keep in mind as you navigate the Autoimmune Protocol. Your primary goals are to maximize your nutrient intake, stabilize your blood sugar, and reduce gut inflammation. But how?

1. Focus on nutrient density.

If you limit yourself only to *removing* all the inflammatory foods from your diet, you have accomplished only half of the job! An autoimmune disease is often accompanied by nutrient deficiencies, so you'll also have to be diligent about *adding* nutrient-rich foods to your menu. Focusing on nutrient density is critical for supporting both the healing process and your immune system.

So, be sure to consume:

A wide variety of vegetables and fruits, including plenty of cruciferous vegetables (such as broccoli, Brussels sprouts, cauliflower, cabbage, collard greens, and kale) and leafy greens

Fermented vegetables

Organ meat

Bone broth

Wild-caught seafood

Grass-fed meat and poultry

2. Consume healthy fats.

Contrary to popular belief, fat isn't always the bad guy! A multitude of bodily processes require fat in order to function optimally, including the building and maintenance of cell membranes, hormone regulation, brain function, and the normal functioning of the nervous and digestive systems. According to an article published by Harvard Medical School, a good rule of thumb is to avoid trans fats, consume saturated fats in moderation, and prioritize good—that is, monounsaturated and polyunsaturated—fats.

So, be sure to consume:

∞ Coconut oil, avocado oil, and olive oil

∞ Lard and tallow

∞ Avocados and olives

∞ Fatty fish

3. Maintain stable blood sugar levels.

Nobody benefits from high blood sugar levels, but the effects are even more detrimental if you suffer from an autoimmune disorder. This is because sugar spikes create a state of constant inflammation in the body, which in turn creates hormonal imbalances and gut dysbiosis, depletes the adrenal glands, and ultimately exacerbates symptoms of autoimmune disease.

So, you should:

∞ Avoid eating sugary breakfasts. Instead, consume a balanced meal in the morning, including a source of protein, healthy fats, and vegetables.

∞ Eat fruit in moderation (maximum 20 grams per day, which represents about two servings).

∞ Limit your consumption of high-glycemic foods, such as dried fruit, fruit juice, natural sweeteners (honey, maple syrup, etc.), AIP-friendly treats, and coconut products (except coconut oil).

∞ Pair high-carb foods (if you are eating them) with fiber and/or protein to slow down the absorption of sugar into the bloodstream.

4. Avoid trigger foods.

One of the chief purposes of the initial elimination phase of AIP is to give your body a "time-out" so that it gets a chance to heal and restore proper gut health. When you remove all the trigger foods from your diet, you slowly break the inflammation/autoimmune flare cycle. This, in turn, will help restore the integrity of the gut lining and improve nutrient absorption.

For these reasons, be sure to avoid all the foods on the Foods to Avoid list (page 18). You will get to reintroduce a lot of these foods later on in the process, during the reintroduction phase, following the step-by-step process described on page 13. Believe me, I know how hard it can be to follow a restricted diet, especially when it gets in the way of old habits. Be strong, though! Committing to AIP 100 percent will be worth it, I promise.

Food Lists

Here are some handy lists with all the foods you should eat and those you should avoid on the Autoimmune Protocol. Make copies of these and keep them in your kitchen and in your handbag, backpack, or briefcase so that you can refer to them quickly when you're grocery shopping. (Important note: When shopping, do not buy dried products from bulk bins to avoid cross-contamination.)

Foods to Eat	
VEGETABLES	artichoke, arugula, asparagus, beet, bok choy, broccoli, Brussels sprouts, butternut squash, cabbage, carrot, cauliflower, celeriac, celery, chard, collard greens, cucumber, daikon, dandelion, endive, fennel, jicama, kale, kohlrabi, leek, lettuce, mushroom, mustard greens, Napa cabbage, okra, onion, parsnip, pumpkin, radicchio, radish, rhubarb, rutabaga, seaweed (such as dulse, nori, and wakame), shallot, spinach, summer squash, sweet potato, taro, turnip, watercress, water chestnuts, winter squash, yam, yuca, zucchini
HERBS AND SPICES	basil leaf, bay leaf, chamomile, chives, cilantro, cinnamon, cloves, dill, fennel leaf, garlic, ginger, lavender, lemongrass, mace, marjoram, mint, oregano leaf, parsley, rosemary, saffron, sage, savory, sea salt, tarragon, thyme, turmeric, vanilla bean (but not the seeds)
FRUIT	apple, apricot, avocado, banana, blackberry, blueberry, cantaloupe, cherry, clementine, coconut, cranberry, date, fig, grape, grapefruit, guava, honeydew, huckleberry, kiwi, lemon, lime, mango, nectarine, olives, orange, papaya, peach, pear, persimmon, pineapple, plantain, plum, pomegranate, raspberry, strawberry, tangerine, watermelon
MEAT	beef, bison, chicken, duck, elk, lamb, mutton, pork, rabbit, turkey, venison, yak
ORGAN MEAT	bone broth, gizzard, heart, kidney, liver, tongue
FISH	anchovies, bass, carp, catfish, cod, haddock, halibut, herring, mackerel, mahi-mahi, monkfish, salmon, sardines, snapper, sole, swordfish, tilapia, trout, tuna
SHELLFISH	clams, crab, crawfish, lobster, mussels, octopus, oysters, prawns, scallops, shrimp, squid
FERMENTS	kombucha, kvass, lacto-fermented fruits and vegetables, sauerkraut, water kefir
FATS	avocado oil, bacon fat, coconut oil, duck fat, lard (rendered pork back or kidney fat), olive oil, palm oil, palm shortening, tallow (rendered fat from beef or lamb)
SWEETENERS	coconut sugar, coconut syrup, dates, dried fruit, honey, maple sugar, maple syrup, molasses

Foods to Consume in Moderation

green and black tea, fructose (maximum 20 grams per day), salt (use mineral-rich salts), AIP treats and baked goods, coconut products, natural sweeteners, moderate- to high-glycemic fruits and vegetables

Foods to Avoid

GRAINS	amaranth, barley, buckwheat, bulgur, corn, farro, kamut, millet, oats, quinoa, rice, rye, sorghum, spelt, teff, wheat
BEANS AND LEGUMES	adzuki beans, black beans, black-eyed peas, calico beans, cannellini beans, chickpeas, fava beans, Great Northern beans, green beans, kidney beans, lentils, lima beans, navy beans, peanuts, peas, pinto beans, split peas, red beans, soybeans (including soy products), sugar snap peas, white beans
NIGHTSHADES	ashwagandha, bell peppers, eggplant, goji berries, ground cherries, jalapeño peppers, potatoes, tobacco, tomatillos, tomatoes (see also spices derived from nightshades)
EGGS	chicken eggs, duck eggs, goose eggs, quail eggs
DAIRY	butter, butter oil, buttermilk, cheese, cottage cheese, cream, cream cheese, frozen yogurt, ghee, goat cheese, goat milk, ice cream, kefir, milk, sour cream, whey, whey protein, yogurt
NUTS AND SEEDS	almonds, Brazil nuts, cashews, chestnuts, chia, cocoa, coffee, flax, hazelnuts, hemp, macadamias, pecans, pine nuts, pistachios, pumpkin seeds, sesame seeds, sunflower seeds (including flours, butters, and oils derived from nuts and seeds)
FATS	canola oil, corn oil, cottonseed oil, palm kernel oil, peanut oil, safflower oil, soybean oil, sunflower oil
HERBS AND SPICES	allspice, anise seed, caraway, cardamom, cayenne pepper*, celery seed, chili pepper flakes*, chili powder*, coriander seed, cumin, curry, dill seed, fennel seed, fenugreek, juniper, mustard seed, nutmeg, paprika*, pepper (all kinds), poppy seed, red pepper*, sesame seed, star anise, sumac, vanilla seeds *spices derived from nightshades
OTHER	alcohol, bee pollen, chlorella, emulsifiers, food additives, food chemicals, maca, processed sugars, processed vegetable oils, spirulina, sugar alcohol and nonnutritive sweeteners (including stevia and xylitol), thickeners, NSAID medications (check with your doctor for pain management)

Adding Flavor to Your Meals

AIP beginners sometimes worry that their food will taste bland without the condiments and sauces they're used to. What about ketchup, mayo, mustard, and barbecue sauce? And what can you use to add kick to your meat and vegetables?

Plenty! I have created an entire collection of AIP-friendly basic sauces and dressings (see pages 176 to 185) that I'm sure you'll love. But first, let's take a look at all the **dried herbs and spices** allowed during the AIP elimination phase. You can find these in the Foods to Eat list on page 17, and you should make full use of them! I have a special drawer in my kitchen within easy reach of the stove where I keep all my go-tos. In that drawer you can find these types of herbs and spices:

- French: rosemary, thyme, sage, herbs de Provence, lavender, parsley, tarragon, garlic, onion powder

- Italian: oregano, basil, marjoram, garlic powder

- Holiday baking: cinnamon, ginger, cloves

- Curry: turmeric, ginger, cinnamon, cloves

Aromatic fresh herbs are great to have on hand, too. You can probably grow some of these in your garden or in containers indoors, which will cut down on your grocery bill. Others you might prefer to buy at the grocery store, like I do: These include cilantro, parsley, and basil. To keep your fresh herbs for longer, place the stem ends in a glass or jar partially filled with water and refrigerate.

Fresh turmeric and ginger root are also fantastic flavor boosters. Make sure you peel them first, then grate using a small handheld grater. Throw the rest of the root in a small resealable plastic bag (or glass container) and refrigerate for later use.

Liquid coconut aminos and fish sauce are other ways to add flavor on the fly. I use them primarily for stir-fries and breakfast skillets.

Again, you'll find a wide selection of sauces and dressings in the Basics chapter (pages 176 to 185). Here is what you can look forward to:

- Dressings: Asian Dressing, Mayonnaise, and Vinaigrette

- Sauces: Basil-Cilantro Pesto, Dairy-Free Cheese Sauce, Marinara Sauce, No-Cook BBQ Sauce, Quick Gravy, Teriyaki Sauce, and Tzatziki Dressing

Hungry yet? If so, read on! The next chapter will show you why meal prep is the best way to stay on track with your AIP diet.

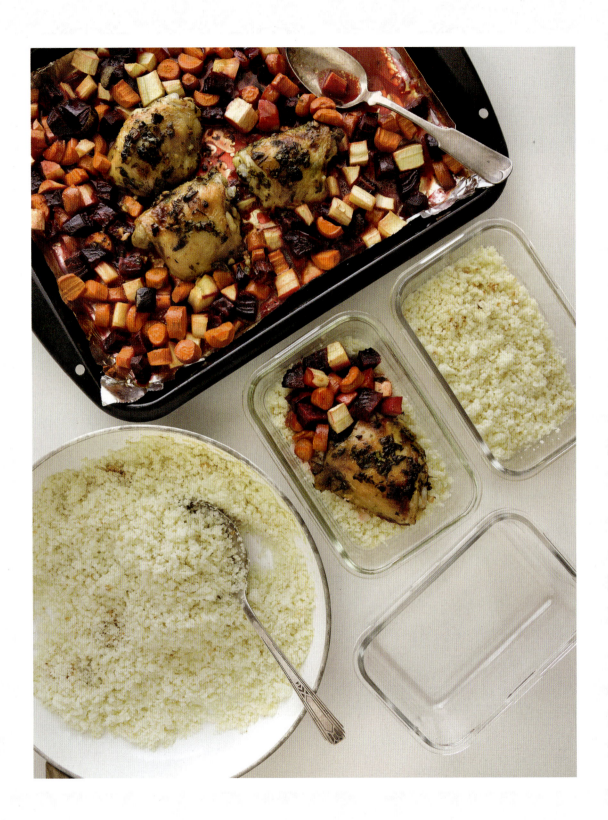

Chapter 2
HOW TO MEAL PREP LIKE A PRO

Knowing which foods to eat and which foods to avoid on the Autoimmune Protocol is a good start, but eating well, day in and day out, while navigating a busy schedule is a whole different ball game! Even under the best of circumstances, eating healthily can be difficult. Add a dash of illness, and it becomes very challenging indeed. But, thanks to meal prep, it doesn't have to be this way. Meal prep is a real game changer. It has numerous benefits and will help you stick to AIP—and achieve your health goals—in the long term.

Here's what meal prep can do for you:

Help you stay on track with your AIP diet. It's so much easier to be successful on the AIP when you are organized and prepare your meals in advance. For a limited time, while your food choices are restricted to the AIP-approved ingredients list (page 17), old quick-fix habits, such as grabbing a slice of pizza or getting fast food, are no longer options. So, taking the time to batch-cook your meals for the rest of the week in a single session is a tremendous help, well worth the initial effort. It's like having your own AIP-approved catering service! When you're ready to eat, all you have to do is reheat your meal, then sit back and enjoy it, knowing that you are nourishing your body with all the nutrients it needs to heal and thrive.

Save time. The batch-cooking session to prep your meals for the week won't take more than two or three hours of work. Plus, it's much more efficient to get all the pots and pans out and cook your meals in a single session than going through the motions of cooking from scratch every night. That means you only have to worry about one big kitchen cleanup! (And if you're lucky, that is a task you can easily delegate to children, spouses, or grateful friends.) Finally, once you get the hang of this whole meal-prep business, you'll breeze through the batch-cooking directions. Practice makes perfect!

Save money and reduce food waste. Meal prep will help you save money in many ways and keeps you in control of your food budget. Operating with a shopping list ensures that you have all the ingredients you need on hand when you are batch-cooking. This means no more dashing to the grocery store to grab last-minute ingredients, which not only wastes time but also puts you at risk of making unhealthy impulse buys. Having a shopping list also means that you won't buy too much of one food, so you won't end up throwing away unused ingredients that have been languishing in the back of the fridge. I don't know about you, but I hate throwing food away. It's one of my pet peeves!

Remove stress from your life. Meal prep means no more last-minute scrambling in the kitchen to find something edible that won't send you into an autoimmune flare! Breakfast becomes an enjoyable moment instead of a rushed affair, and lunch at work is already taken care of. And what about when you're out and about, having a good time with friends, and everyone else is grabbing a pizza? Or when you are back home visiting your family, and no one is eating the same way you do? Well, when you prep your meals in advance, suddenly you don't have to spend any time at all thinking about what you are going to eat. You are free to enjoy the moment because you don't have to make any (tough!) decisions.

Free up your time to engage in other activities. This benefit of meal prepping is all the more critical when you know that healing from an autoimmune disease isn't just about the food you eat (and don't eat). Lifestyle also plays a huge role in your well-being. Once you don't have to cook every single meal from scratch every day, you suddenly have all this free time you can dedicate to enjoyable, health-promoting activities! Now you can kick back and read a book, relax in a yoga class, let off some steam by exercising, or just spend quality time with your family and friends. You're actually adding hours to your day!

How Does Meal Prep Work?

It's easy, and it can be broken down into four main steps.

1. Select the recipes and create your menu.
The first step is to go through your stock of recipes (cookbooks, blogs, Pinterest, etc.) and select the recipes you would like to eat during the week. Then, create your menu for each day. When you're doing this, be mindful of seasonal products and variety. Try to eat a broad range of foods, including different sources of protein (meat/seafood) and high-starch and low-starch vegetables. Include a

versatile salad (that you can quickly turn into a full meal by adding a protein, such as cooked chicken or shrimp). Pay attention to the servings each recipe yields. You may have to adapt the quantities to fit your needs: Are you cooking for just yourself, or a family of four?

2. Make a master list.

Write down a list of all the ingredients and tools you will need to prepare all the recipes in your menu. Cross off from the list the items you already have on hand in your refrigerator, freezer, and pantry. Purchase all the ingredients you'll need and store them appropriately until you are ready for your batch-cooking session. Ideally, you'll want to do your shopping the day before your batch-cooking session to ensure your ingredients are as fresh as possible. Have you noticed that produce (or meat, poultry, and seafood) stays fresh longer at one particular store compared to others? The farm-to-consumer transit time may vary greatly, and the longer it takes for fresh vegetables and fruit to reach you, the more nutrients they lose. Buying from local producers (and in season) will maximize the nutritional value of your ingredients.

3. Set up your batch-cooking session.

All it takes is a little planning. First, schedule a day that works for you. For most people, Sunday would be the obvious choice, with the shopping done on Saturday. Each batch-cooking session shouldn't take more than half a day, including kitchen cleanup. Then, plan your cooking session. I recommend reading through the batch-cooking directions at least once before you start cooking, especially to make sure you have all the tools required.

Here are a couple more tips:

- Some menus call for bone broth. Unless you have found a reliable source of store-bought, AIP-compliant bone broth, you will have to prepare your own in advance (see page 180 for slow cooker and pressure cooker directions).

- Make sure you allow enough time for your frozen ingredients to thaw.

- Have all your containers clean and ready with their corresponding lids!

4. Game day! Cook, assemble, store.

Your batch-cooking session should go pretty smoothly if you have gone through the preparations in the previous three steps. I recommend starting early in the day. That way, you have plenty of time to cook without feeling rushed, to let the food cool completely before storing, and to clean up your kitchen and tools.

Tips for Proper Food Storage

Meal planning and batch-cooking have lots of benefits: For instance, they help you eat healthier and save money and time. But how to keep your meals fresh and tasty throughout the week? You've worked hard to prepare nutritious meals; now you'll want to make sure they stay fresh for as long as possible. Follow these simple tips on safe handling and storage of leftovers and cooked foods.

- Purchase the freshest ingredients possible and schedule your batch-cooking session promptly after purchasing.

- Don't overcook your food. Overcooked food makes for poor leftovers; proteins dry out, and vegetables become mushy. I provide cooking time, target temperatures, and visual cues in each recipe to help ensure each meal is perfectly cooked.

- Once your meal has been cooked, divide it into smaller portions right away and store them in glass containers. Allow the food to cool first, then close each container with an airproof and leakproof lid. This will prevent loss of flavor and moisture.

- Refrigerate (or freeze) food within 2 hours of cooking to avoid bacteria growth. You may speed the cooling process (especially recommended during hot summer months) by placing the closed containers in a bath of ice-cold water before storing.

- If you decide to freeze your meals, label and date the containers. Consume these meals within 4 months.

- Make sure your refrigerator is set to the proper temperature (between 32°F and 40°F [0°C and 4.5°C] maximum). Store your meals on the top and middle shelves, leaving space in between for the cold air to move freely and consistently. The lower shelf, which is the coldest, is better suited to raw proteins, eggs, and dairy. Use the crisp drawers at the very bottom of the fridge to store fresh vegetables and fruit.

- Keep the containers refrigerated until you are ready to eat. If you are traveling, or are on the go or at the office, keep your meals cold in a portable insulated cooler, along with an ice pack.

Tips for Reheating Your Meals

Now you know how to handle and store your cooked meals, but did you know that the way you thaw (if frozen) and reheat your meals also plays an essential role in preserving flavor and preventing bacteria growth? Here's how to make sure you get the best from your frozen meals.

FOR PREVIOUSLY FROZEN FOOD

Most of the recipes in this cookbook are freezer friendly (unless otherwise noted), so you always have the option to freeze part or all of your meals after your batch-cooking session. In a perfect world, you would never forget to thaw your meals a day or two in advance. But we all know that life gets in the way, and some days you might forget to take your container out of the freezer. If this happens, remember that it is safe to reheat frozen food without thawing it first (either in a saucepan, in the oven, or in the microwave), but I don't recommend this as a rule. That's because it takes a long time to reheat, needs a lot of supervision, and it seems to leach moisture from the food. Thus, I find that setting a reminder on my smartphone helps me remember to take meals out of the freezer a day or two in advance.

HOW TO SAFELY THAW A FROZEN MEAL

Frozen food is safe as long as it stays frozen (at 40°F [4.5°C] or lower). Once you initiate the thawing process, bacteria will start to develop. As a rule, never let your frozen meals sit around at room temperature on the kitchen countertop for an extended period of time. This is because harmful bacteria develop between 40°F and 140°F (4.5°C and 60°C), increasing the risk of foodborne illnesses. Don't be alarmed, though: There are several ways to safely thaw your frozen meals, depending on how much time you have.

- **Refrigerator:** Allowing the frozen meal to thaw slowly in the fridge is by far the best and safest route. The temperature inside the refrigerator will prevent any bacteria from growing. This requires some planning in advance, though, as it may take anywhere from 24 to 48 hours for the meal to be fully thawed.

- **Cold water:** This technique is a bit more labor-intensive, but it's still a good option if you need to consume your meal on the same day. Submerge the container (with a leakproof lid) in a bowl of cold water and change the water every 30 minutes. This also works directly in the sink. Even though you may be tempted to speed the process, don't use hot water to do this. It may take several hours to fully thaw your meal this way.

- **Microwave:** If you are short on time, using the DEFROST function of your microwave is also a safe option for thawing your frozen meal. Before you start, make sure your meal is in a microwave-safe container, though (see page 26 for more information). Use a cover to retain moisture and avoid splattering. Also, it's a good idea to stir your meal a few times during the process to ensure uniform thawing. Continue until the food is piping hot and ready to eat.

HOW TO REHEAT YOUR MEALS

The name of the game here is slow and steady. Avoid rushing or using scorchingly high temperatures in order to preserve flavor and moisture and keep your food tasting great and looking appealing. See pages 32 to 33 for more container types to make sure yours is suitable for a specific heating method.

- **Oven and toaster oven:** This is a simple way to reheat your meal slowly. Set the temperature to no higher than 350°F (180°C or gas mark 4) and cover the container with aluminum foil to lock in moisture.

- **Microwave:** Fast and oh-so-convenient, this method is best suited for meals with a higher moisture content, such as soups, stews, stir-fries, and skillets. I like to drizzle my leftovers with a little bit of oil before microwaving. Oh, and don't forget to cover the container to prevent the moisture from escaping! Finally, it also helps to stir the contents at least once during cooking to ensure that everything is heated through.

- **Stovetop:** Stick to low and medium temperatures, and stir the food regularly. It's also a good idea to add some liquid so that the food won't stick to the bottom of the saucepan or skillet. I recommend using olive oil, avocado oil, coconut oil, chicken broth, or even water. As with microwaving, cover with a lid to retain heat and moisture.

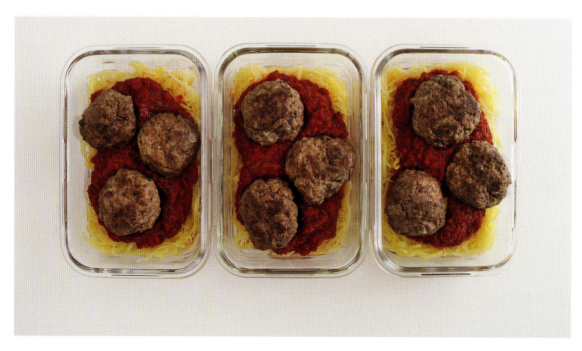

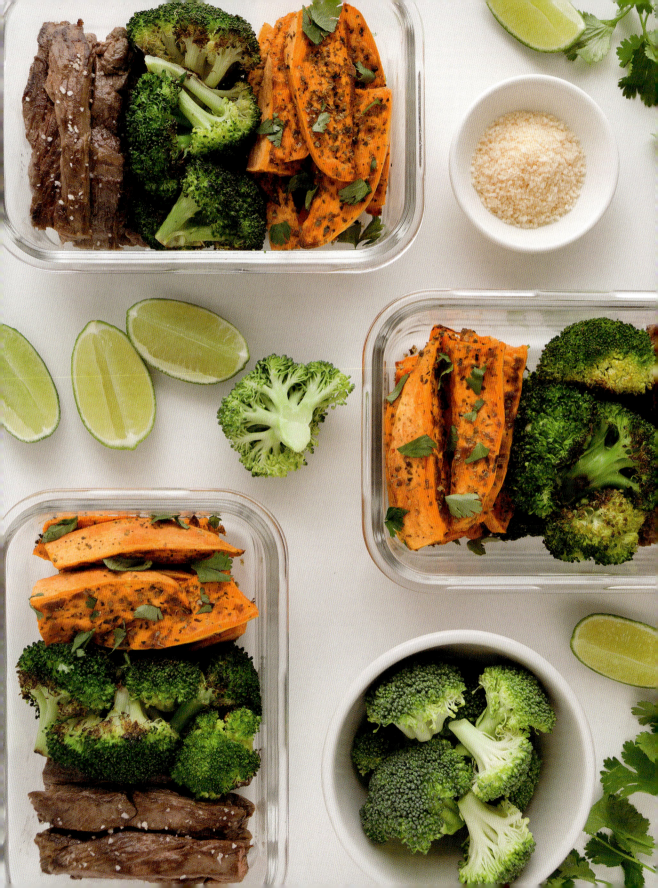

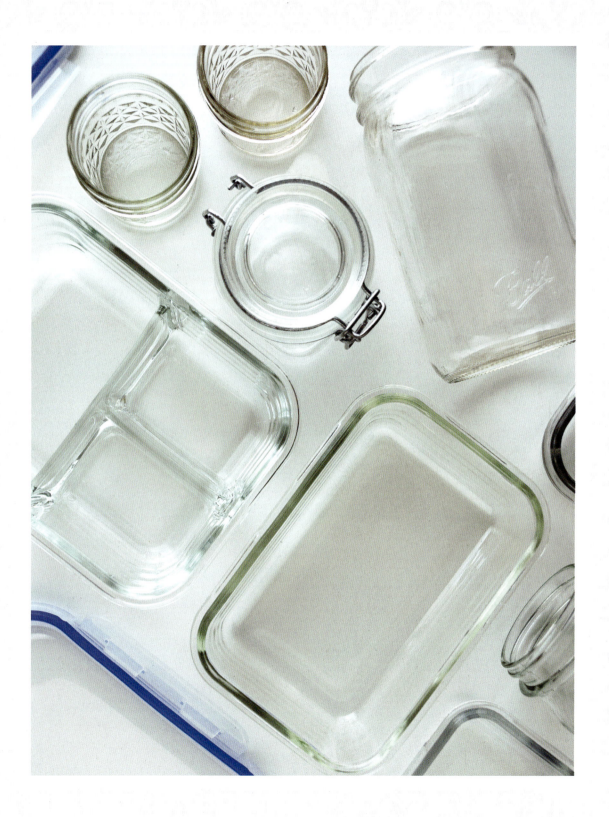

Chapter 3
GETTING READY TO MEAL PREP

N ow it's time to assemble your tools! The next steps are to make sure you have all the essential ingredients, equipment and supplies, and storage containers that will help make meal prep even easier.

AIP Ingredients

First, stock your pantry. Here's a list of all the pantry items you'll need to prepare all the recipes in this book. (You may already have lots of them!)

Apple cider vinegar: An amber-colored vinegar made from fermented apple juice with a wonderful, zingy, energizing smell and taste. In its purest form, ACV may appear cloudy, thanks to strands of good-for-your-gut enzymes and health-promoting probiotics.

Arrowroot flour/starch: This white powder is an ideal replacement for traditional cornstarch. Reach for it whenever you need to thicken a sauce or make gravy. Since it's super-light, I also mix it with other, heavier AIP flours to achieve a lighter texture in my baked goods. Handle with care: it tends to fly up into the air as soon as it gets out of the bag!

Baking powder: Used to lighten the texture and increase the volume of baked goods. Be aware that store-bought versions often contain cornstarch and/or aluminum, which are not AIP friendly. But you can get around this by making your own baking powder. Just mix 2 tablespoons (16 g) cream of tartar with 1 tablespoon (8 g) baking soda and store in an airtight container.

Balsamic vinegar: A dark brown vinegar made from white grape juice with a rich, sweet, complex flavor. Use it for dressings or my nightshade-free Marinara Sauce (page 183).

Blackstrap molasses (unsulfured): Made from crushed sugarcane, this dark brown syrup has a rich and distinctive smoky flavor. It is the secret ingredient in my No-Cook BBQ Sauce (page 184)!

Carob powder (roasted): This brown powder is used in place of cocoa powder in AIP baking. I prefer the roasted kind: It blends more smoothly with liquids. Try mixing it with hot coconut milk and a dash of maple syrup or honey for a cup of AIP-friendly hot chocolate!

Cassava flour: This thick, high-fiber flour is made from peeled, ground cassava root and is very popular in AIP cuisine. You can use it alone—to make tortillas, for example—or blend it with other AIP-friendly flours when baking.

Coconut aminos: Similar in taste and color to soy sauce, coconut aminos is made from the sap of the coconut tree (but doesn't taste like coconut at all!). I use it all the time: in dressings, marinades, and stir-fries. It's great for adding a flavor boost to almost all your savory dishes.

Coconut flour: Here's another dense, high-fiber flour. This one has a slightly sweet taste,

so it's often used in AIP baking. It acts like a sponge and absorbs all the liquids it comes into contact with, so use it sparingly.

Coconut milk (unsweetened): Look for the canned version, and read the label carefully to make sure no thickening agents or emulsifiers are hiding in the ingredients list! Coconut milk is rich and creamy, very much like traditional heavy cream, so it's widely used in AIP cuisine for sauces and desserts alike. Pro tip: Sometimes a recipe may call for coconut cream. Make your own coconut cream by scooping the creamy top from a can of full-fat coconut milk that has been refrigerated for at least 24 hours.

Coconut oil: This creamy white oil is a staple in my AIP kitchen and is safe to use at higher temperatures (over 350°F [180°C or gas mark 4]). It's usually a solid but will liquify if you live in a hot climate. (You can use it topically, too: Rub a little into your hands for instantly soft, smooth skin!)

Fish sauce: A dark amber liquid made from fermented black anchovy, this sauce packs plenty of savory flavor! Look for it in the Shrimp Pad Thai recipe (page 88), or use it any time a dish needs an umami kick.

Gelatin powder (unflavored): This grainy, sand-colored protein powder has the unique property of turning liquids into gel. It's the secret ingredient used to make those fun gummies that are so popular in the AIP community (see Pomegranate Gummies, page

169). Gelatin is also used as an egg replacer when baking.

Nutritional yeast (not fortified): This inactive form of yeast is high in protein and presents itself in the form of yellow flakes or powder. It has a unique and distinctive cheesy flavor and is used in AIP cuisine to prepare faux cheese sauce (see my Dairy-Free Cheese Sauce, page 182).

Oils: Avocado oil, coconut oil, and olive oil turn up everywhere in this cookbook. Use olive oil for salad dressings and cooking at low temperatures (350°F [180°C or gas mark 4] and lower), and reserve avocado oil and coconut oil for oven baking or roasting, or when cooking over medium heat on the stovetop.

Palm shortening: This thick and creamy shortening, which is solid at room temperature, is often used for baking in AIP cuisine as a replacement for traditional shortening or butter. Look for an eco-friendly, sustainable source if possible.

Tigernut flour: You'd be forgiven for thinking that this is a nut flour, but tigernuts are actually small, round root vegetables! When ground into powder, tigernuts yield a light brown flour, sometimes grainy, with a slightly nutty flavor. I love to blend it with other AIP flours when baking.

Make sure you have the following staples on hand, too: honey, maple syrup, black olives, capers, unsweetened applesauce, pumpkin puree, canned tuna, and unsweetened shredded coconut.

Also, when you're grocery shopping, always read the nutrition information labels carefully to avoid non-AIP-compliant ingredients—especially when you're buying canned or packaged goods.

Equipment and Supplies

You won't have to purchase any special or expensive tools to start the Autoimmune Protocol. Like me, you'll be able to keep things as simple as possible, minimizing time and expense. I choose to allocate the larger part of my food budget to quality ingredients, such as organic, grass-fed meats or wild-caught seafood, rather than to kitchen gadgets. (The fact that I don't enjoy all the kitchen gadget cleanup may also play a significant role in this decision!)

To get started, you'll need all the basic tools found in any kitchen, such as:

- chef's knife and paring knife
- cutting board
- measuring cups and spoons
- slotted spoon or spatula
- vegetable peeler
- mixing bowls
- pots and pans (including a stockpot)
- parchment paper, aluminum foil, 1-gallon (3.6 L) resealable plastic bags

I also recommend getting *two large rimmed baking sheets (12 x 17 inches [30.5 x 43 cm])* and *one large nonstick skillet (at least 11 inches [28 cm] wide)*, even if you are cooking only for yourself. Because you're going to be batch-cooking in large quantities, you need tools that will allow you to cook, bake, or fry several meals all at once.

You will also need these inexpensive and less conventional tools (you'll get a lot of use out of them, I promise). As for the electrical items, don't feel obliged to get the fancy, top-of-the-line versions. The basic models you'll find at your local home goods store will work just fine.

- vegetable spiralizer, for transforming just about any vegetable into "noodles"

- handheld potato masher, for making vegetable mash

- slow cooker (6 quart [5.4 L])

- blenders (a handheld blender for soups and a tabletop blender for sauces and batters)

- food processor with an S-blade and a shredding disk

- electric pressure cooker (such as a 6-quart [5.4 L] Instant Pot. You will need this only for two recipes in this book; see the One-Pot Meal Plan, pages 149–146)

Some meal plans will have you cook different meals at the same time in the oven. For

this reason, make sure you have at least two racks in your oven to work with.

And, of course, you will need containers to store all your meals!

Choosing the Right Containers

For each batch-cooking session in this cookbook, you will need to prepare at least fifteen containers to store your breakfasts, lunches, and dinners. **Each meal best fits a 28- to 30-ounce (784 to 840 g) container size.** You will also need at least five smaller containers for your snacks.

You have lots of options when it comes to food containers: glass, metal, plastic, jars, with or without compartments. Let's have a look at the pros and cons of each option so that you can decide what's best for you.

GLASS CONTAINERS

These are by far my first choice when it comes to food storage containers. Yes, they tend to be heavier, and they are breakable, but they're so convenient!

These containers are freezer, oven, microwave, and dishwasher safe. (Plastic lids, however, may warp when put in the dishwasher.) This means that you don't have to transfer the food to a plate to heat up your meal (unless you prefer to, of course). But you do need to remove the lids when reheating your food (unless they come with built-in venting openings), and I recommend washing them by hand in warm soapy water.

Choose a design with airtight and water-tight locking lids. Because they prevent contact with air, these locking mechanisms ensure that food stays fresh for longer and prevent food spillage and leaks, too.

I prefer rectangular containers, as they fit better in the cupboards, freezer, and fridge. (Pro tip: Always store your empty containers with the lids on! I spent years diving into my drawers searching for matching tops until I finally adopted this simple trick.)

You can also use glass jars with metal lids. These come in all sizes and are particularly suited to stews, soups, and salads. I like to use small 4- to 8-ounce (112 to 227 g) glass jars to store all manner of snacks (see Blueberry Mousse, page 159, and Carrot Cake Muffins, page 48).

METAL CONTAINERS

For style and durability, nothing beats metal containers. They're virtually unbreakable, dishwasher safe, and much lighter than their glass counterparts.

Make sure you select food-grade stainless steel containers. Some models come with leakproof lids, while others have only a lid that latches on with a clip. The latter is not suitable for meals that contain a lot of liquid, such as stews and soups.

Also, keep in mind that metal containers are not suitable for microwaves (and aren't likely to be suitable for oven use, either).

PLASTIC CONTAINERS

Inexpensive and disposable, plastic containers can be found pretty much anywhere, even at your local grocery store. Major online retailers also sell them in large multipacks at very competitive prices. Look for BPA-free food-grade plastic.

Most of these plastic containers are freezer and microwave safe, but can't be used in the oven. Wash them in warm soapy water, although you might not be able to get rid of lingering food smells (and tastes) if you reuse them often.

Plastic might be a good option if you are on the go or traveling and won't be able to go back home anytime soon. But please be considerate of the environment and recycle plastic containers instead of throwing them out with the regular trash.

Whether you get food containers with built-in compartments is entirely up to you. I don't care much for them, but I can see how they would be handy for storing small snacks separately, such as cheese, grapes, and crackers, or if you don't like the different components of a meal touching one another.

How to Use the Meal Plans in This Book

Are you ready to start meal prepping? Begin by selecting your meal plan. Each meal plan in this cookbook has a specific theme, making it easy for you to accommodate your dietary needs (and your current mood!). Refer to the short introduction at the beginning of each plan to get a quick overview of the lineup of dishes.

Each meal plan is designed to feed one adult for five days, including breakfast, lunch, dinner, and a nutritious snack. This leaves you two days in which you can cook fresh or eat out. If you are cooking for a bigger crowd, increase the ingredients on the ready-made shopping lists to fit your needs. The cooking times will remain the same, but you will probably have to execute the cooking directions in multiple batches. If you end up with leftovers, you may freeze them for later use. All the recipes in this cookbook are freezer friendly unless otherwise noted.

Each week, in addition to the meal plan, you'll need to prepare some bone broth. The recipe on page 180 will give you slow cooker and pressure cooker directions. Some weeks you'll need bone broth to prepare the recipes included in your meal plan. (Don't worry about forgetting: I remind you of this at the beginning of each batch-cooking session.) What you

don't use in recipes, reserve and drink a little every day as part of your gut-healing routine.

If the portions are too big for you to eat in one sitting, keep the leftovers to eat between meals as snacks. Or, if you find yourself hungry between meals, complement your meals with AIP-compliant snacks, such as avocados, canned sardines, olives, prosciutto, fruit, or coconut milk yogurt. You may also supplement each meal with a side salad (get a ready-made salad mix at your local store) and some dressing (see the Basics chapter, pages 176 to 186, for dressings and sauces).

Once you have selected your meal plan for the week, make a copy of the shopping list, get the ingredients, and follow the instructions for the batch-cooking session. It's that simple!

A final note before you get started: I designed the batch-cooking sessions in this cookbook to take the least amount of time to complete. For this reason, in some meal plans you may have to perform different tasks from different recipes simultaneously. To make sure everything goes smoothly, read through the directions at least once before starting to cook. This is the best way to avoid unwelcome last-minute surprises, like discovering that you're missing ingredients or tools!

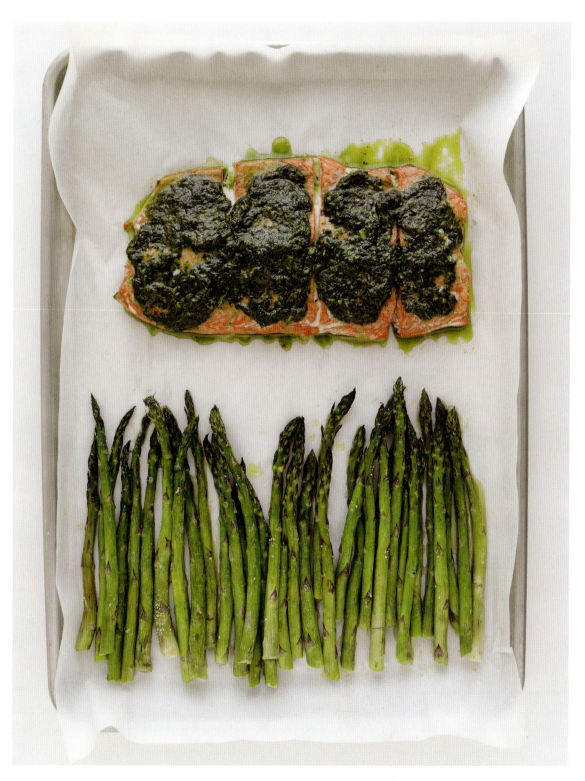

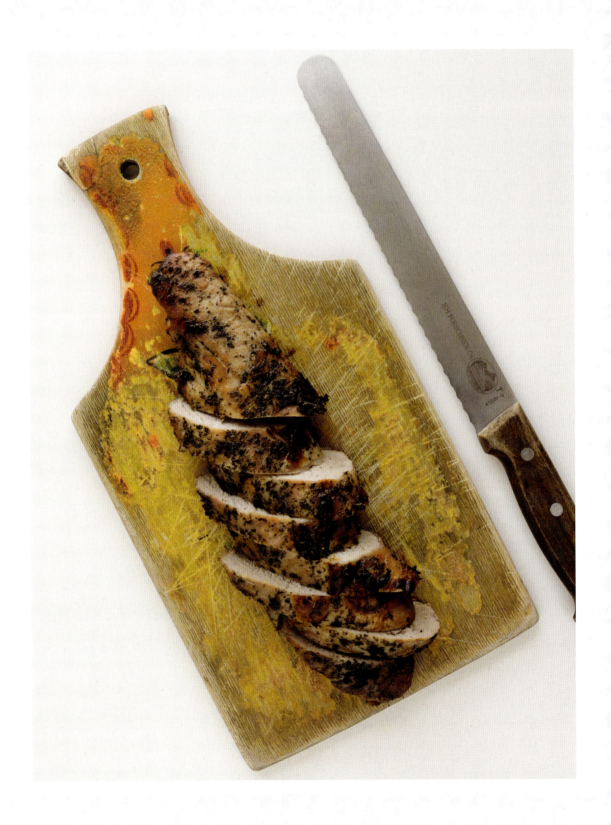

Chapter 4
COMFORT FOOD MEAL PLAN

· · · · · · · · · · · ·

If you're craving comfort food, you've come to the right place! This menu of whole-some, satisfying meals will keep you sated and your energy levels up—even on days when you can't afford to be anything less than 100 percent. It's full of easily digestible proteins plus plenty of both high- and low-starch vegetables for maximum nutrient intake.

Cuban Mojo Chicken with Cauliflower Rice and Roasted Root Vegetables is a colorful Cuban-inspired dish featuring a perfectly seasoned, sweet and spicy mari-nade, and the **Herbed Pork Tenderloin with Sweet Potato and Creamed Kale** is so easy to prepare that it's sure to become one of your favorite weekday meals. (Plus, you won't feel guilty diving into the sweet potato mash because it comes with a whole serving of leafy greens!)

Italian Meatballs are a classic, and mine are served with Baked Spaghetti Squash instead of traditional pasta, which makes for a much healthier meal. And wait until you taste the nightshade-free Marinara Sauce: You'll want to smear it on everything!

For lunch, there's a refreshing **Niçoise Salad**; it's portable, too, so it's a great option whether you're at home, at the office, or on the go.

What about snack time? A healthy portion of shredded carrots plays hide-and-seek in my good-for-you **Carrot Cake Muffins**. Enjoy one whenever midday cravings strike!

Share extra portions with family or friends, or save them for the weekends. It's easy, because all three cooked meals in this menu are suitable for freezing.

Kitchen note: Make sure you have 1⅓ cups (315 ml) of chicken Bone Broth available when you start the batch-cooking session.

	BREAKFAST	LUNCH	DINNER	SNACK
DAY 1	Cuban Mojo Chicken	Niçoise Salad	Herbed Pork Tenderloin	Carrot Cake Muffin
DAY 2	Italian Meatballs	Niçoise Salad	Cuban Mojo Chicken	Carrot Cake Muffin
DAY 3	Herbed Pork Tenderloin	Cuban Mojo Chicken	Italian Meatballs	Carrot Cake Muffin
DAY 4	Cuban Mojo Chicken	Niçoise Salad	Herbed Pork Tenderloin	Carrot Cake Muffin
DAY 5	Italian Meatballs	Niçoise Salad	Herbed Pork Tenderloin	Carrot Cake Muffin

EXTRA SERVINGS: 1 Italian Meatballs

Shopping List

PRODUCE

Juice of 1 lime

Juice of 1 orange + ⅓ cup (80 ml) freshly
squeezed orange juice

3 cloves garlic

8 radishes

2 tablespoons (30 ml) lemon juice

3 tablespoons (30 g) finely diced red onion

¼ cup (4 g) chopped fresh cilantro

½ cup (55 g) shredded carrot

½ pound (227 g) parsnips

1 cucumber (¾ pound [340 g])

1 zucchini (¾ pound [340 g])

2 (8-ounce [227 g]) bunches kale

1 pound (454 g) carrots

2 pounds (908 g) beets

1 head cauliflower (2 pounds [908 g])

2½ pounds (1135 g) sweet potatoes +
1 (10-ounce [280 g]) sweet potato

1 spaghetti squash (3 pounds [1362 g])

MEAT/SEAFOOD

2 (5-ounce [140 g]) cans tuna

1⅓ cups (315 ml) chicken Bone Broth (page 180)

1 pound (454 g) ground beef

1 pound (454 g) ground pork

1 pork tenderloin (1 pound [454 g])

4 chicken thighs (1½ pounds [680 g])

HERBS AND SPICES

Pinch ground cloves

½ teaspoon dried cilantro

½ teaspoon ground cinnamon

½ teaspoon ginger powder

1½ teaspoons garlic powder

3 teaspoons (2 g) dried marjoram

3½ teaspoons (2 g) dried basil

3½ teaspoons (2 g) dried oregano

PANTRY ITEMS

¼ teaspoon baking powder

½ tablespoon unflavored gelatin powder

4 teaspoons (25 g) honey

2 tablespoons (30 ml) balsamic vinegar

2 tablespoons (20 g) capers

2 tablespoons (16 g) coconut flour

3 tablespoons (45 ml) coconut aminos

¼ cup (60 g) unsweetened applesauce

¼ cup (60 ml) maple syrup

¼ cup (60 g) palm shortening

⅓ cup (40 g) cassava flour

⅓ cup (40 g) tigernut flour

½ cup (50 g) sliced black olives

1 cup (240 ml) full-fat coconut milk

OTHER

Coconut oil

Extra-virgin olive oil

Sea salt

Equipment and Tools

15 containers for meals + 5 containers for snacks
    (see pages 32 to 33)

6- or 12-cup muffin pan

aluminum foil

baking dish

can opener

cooling rack

cutting board

foil baking cups

food processor (with S-blade)

large skillet (at least 11 inches [28 cm] wide)

measuring cups and spoons

mixing bowls

paring knife, serrated knife, chef's knife

potato masher

pots and pans

rimmed roasting pan (broiler pan style)

rubber spatula

vegetable peeler

vegetable spiralizer

whisk

wooden spoon

Batch-Cooking Directions

1. Reminder: *The morning before*, thaw the meat, if frozen. *The day before*, complete steps 1 and 2 of the **Cuban Mojo Chicken** (page 41) and refrigerate. Make sure you have 1⅓ cups (315 ml) of chicken **Bone Broth** (page 180) on hand. Prepare your containers.

2. Preheat the oven to 375°F (190°C or gas mark 5) and place the rack in the middle of the oven. Complete steps 1 through 6 of the **Carrot Cake Muffins** (page 48). Set a timer for 20 minutes.

3. While the muffins are baking, complete steps 3 through 5 of the **Cuban Mojo Chicken** (page 41), but don't start cooking it yet.

4. When the timer rings for the muffins, transfer them to a cooling rack. Increase the oven heat to 400°F (200°C or gas mark 6) and start cooking the chicken and root vegetables. Set a timer for 40 minutes.

5. Meanwhile, prepare and cook the **Cauliflower Rice** (page 177). Also prepare the **Spaghetti Squash** for the **Italian Meatballs** (page 179), following the oven directions in step 2, but don't start cooking yet.

6. When the timer rings for the chicken and root vegetables, remove them from the oven and start cooking the **Spaghetti Squash** (page 179, step 2). Set a timer for 30 minutes. Now assemble the **Cuban Mojo Chicken** in the containers.

7. Complete steps 2 through 5 of the **Italian Meatballs** (page 44), and assemble.

8. Increase the oven heat to 425°F (220°C or gas mark 7). Complete the **Herbed Pork Tenderloin** (page 43), steps 2 through 5, and assemble.

9. Finish your batch-cooking session with the **Niçoise Salad** (page 47), steps 1 through 3, and assemble.

10. Don't forget to store the muffins cooling on the rack!

CUBAN MOJO CHICKEN *with* CAULIFLOWER RICE *and* ROASTED ROOT VEGETABLES

To make your batch-cooking session go faster, complete step 1 of this recipe the day before and let the chicken marinate overnight. Alternatively, you can prepare step 1 several days in advance and freeze. Thaw completely before using.

Prep time:
25 minutes + marinating time
Cook time:
45 minutes
Yield:
4 servings

4 chicken thighs, about 1½ pounds (680 g)

FOR THE MARINADE:

¼ cup (60 ml) olive oil

Juice of 1 lime

Juice of 1 orange

¼ cup (4 g) chopped fresh cilantro

3 cloves garlic, minced

2 teaspoons (1 g) dried oregano

¾ teaspoon sea salt

½ pound (227 g) beets

½ pound (227 g) carrots

½ pound (227 g) parsnips

Sea salt

1 recipe Cauliflower Rice (page 177)

1. Two hours in advance, or the night before, pat the chicken dry and place in a resealable plastic bag.

2. To make the marinade, in a small bowl, combine the ingredients for the marinade and mix well. Pour over the chicken and seal the bag, turning it over a few times to coat the chicken completely. Refrigerate for at least 2 hours, massaging the chicken in the bag a few times during the marinating process.

3. Peel and dice the beets, carrots, and parsnips.

4. Preheat the oven to 400°F (200°C or gas mark 6) and place the rack in the middle. Line a rimmed roasting pan with aluminum foil.

5. Remove the chicken from the bag, reserving the marinade. Place the marinated chicken in the center of the roasting pan, skin-side up, and spread the beets, carrots, and parsnips around it. Pour over the leftover marinade and sprinkle the root vegetables with salt to taste. Transfer to the oven and bake for 40 to 45 minutes, until the chicken is golden brown and reaches an internal temperature of 165°F (74°C).

6. While the chicken and root vegetables are cooking, prepare the Cauliflower Rice following the directions on page 177.

To assemble: Divide evenly among 4 containers. Place a layer of cauliflower rice at the bottom of each container, then top with a piece of chicken and a quarter of the root vegetables.

Note: Store for up to 5 days in an airtight container in the refrigerator, or freeze for up to 4 months.

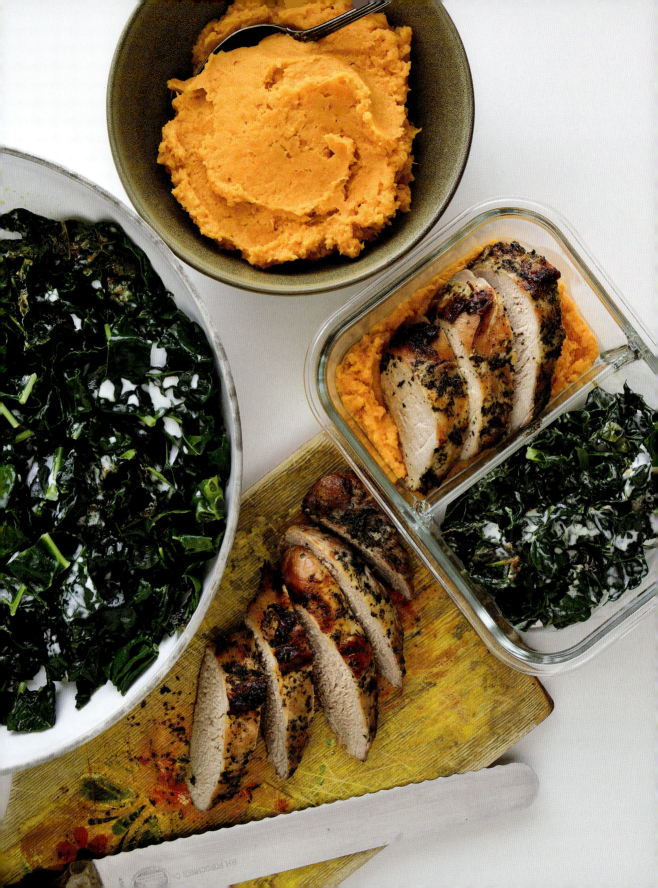

HERBED PORK TENDERLOIN *with* SWEET POTATO MASH *and* CREAMED KALE

Simple, nutritious, and incredibly comforting, this colorful meal deserves a prominent place in your recipe repertoire. Seasoned, perfectly cooked pork tenderloin is surrounded by a rich sweet potato mash and creamy greens. Swap kale for chard or collard greens to vary your source of plant-based nutrients!

Prep time:
20 minutes
Cook time:
30 minutes
Yield:
4 servings

1 pound (454 g) pork tenderloin

3 tablespoons (45 ml) olive oil, divided

1 tablespoon (20 g) honey

½ teaspoon dried basil

½ teaspoon dried cilantro

¼ teaspoon sea salt

1 recipe Sweet Potato Mash (page 184)

2 bunches kale (½ pound [227 g] each)

½ cup (120 ml) full-fat coconut milk

1. Preheat the oven to 425°F (220°C or gas mark 7) and place the rack in the middle.

2. Line a rimmed roasting pan with aluminum foil and place the meat in the center. In a small dish, combine 2 tablespoons (30 ml) of the olive oil with the honey, basil, cilantro, and salt. Pour the mixture over the meat and rub with your fingers to coat. Transfer to the oven and bake for 25 to 30 minutes, basting halfway through, or until the internal temperature reaches 145°F (63°C). When done, remove from the oven and let sit for 10 minutes before slicing.

3. Meanwhile, start making the sweet potato mash following the directions on page 184, steps 1 through 2, and set a timer for 20 minutes.

4. While the meat and potatoes are cooking, remove and discard the woody stems from the kale. Chop the leaves. Heat the remaining 1 tablespoon (15 ml) olive oil in a large skillet over medium heat. Add the kale and ½ cup (120 ml) coconut milk. Cover and cook, stirring occasionally, until tender, about 10 minutes. (You may have to do this in several batches.)

5. When the potatoes are done, finish the sweet potato mash following step 3 on page 184.

To assemble: Divide the sliced meat, mashed sweet potatoes, and creamed kale evenly among 4 containers.

Note: Store for up to 5 days in an airtight container in the refrigerator, or freeze for up to 4 months.

ITALIAN MEATBALLS *with* SPAGHETTI SQUASH *and* MARINARA SAUCE

It's easy to ditch the gluten and enjoy the taste and texture of classic spaghetti and meatballs: just swap your traditional pasta for spaghetti squash noodles! This low-carb squash is rich in dietary fiber, antioxidants, minerals, and vitamins.

Prep time:
25 minutes

Cook time:
35 minutes

Yield:
4 servings

1 recipe Baked Spaghetti Squash (page 179)

1 recipe Marinara Sauce (page 183)

1 pound (454 g) ground beef

1 pound (454 g) ground pork

3 tablespoons (30 g) finely chopped red onion

1 teaspoon dried basil

1 teaspoon dried marjoram

¾ teaspoon salt

½ teaspoon garlic powder

1 tablespoon (15 ml) olive oil

1. Preheat the oven to 400°F (200°C or gas mark 6) and place the rack in the middle. Start cooking the Baked Spaghetti Squash in the oven following the directions on page 179, step 2, and set a timer for 30 minutes.

2. Start making the Marinara Sauce following the directions on page 183, step 1, and set a timer for 30 minutes.

3. Meanwhile, combine the beef, pork, onion, basil, marjoram, salt, and garlic powder in a bowl. Mix thoroughly using your hands and form into 12 meatballs. Heat the olive oil in a large skillet over medium heat and add the meatballs. Cover and fry until cooked through, about 20 minutes, turning them halfway through cooking.

4. Transfer the spaghetti squash to a plate and allow to cool before scraping out the flesh with a fork, making spaghetti noodles.

5. When the vegetables for the Marinara Sauce are done cooking, finish the sauce following the directions in step 2, page 183.

To assemble: Divide the spaghetti squash evenly among 4 containers and top each with a generous serving of Marinara Sauce plus 3 meatballs.

Note: Store for up to 5 days in an airtight container in the refrigerator, or freeze for up to 4 months.

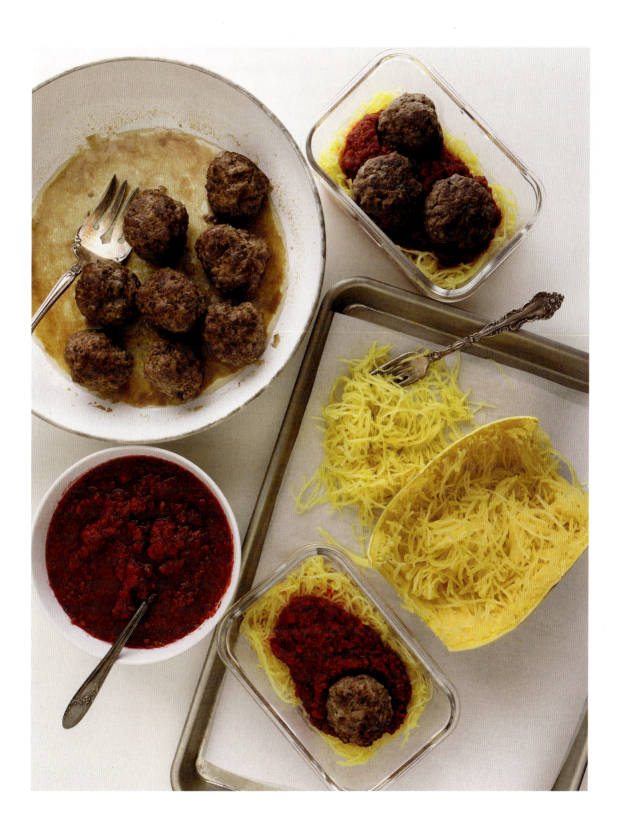

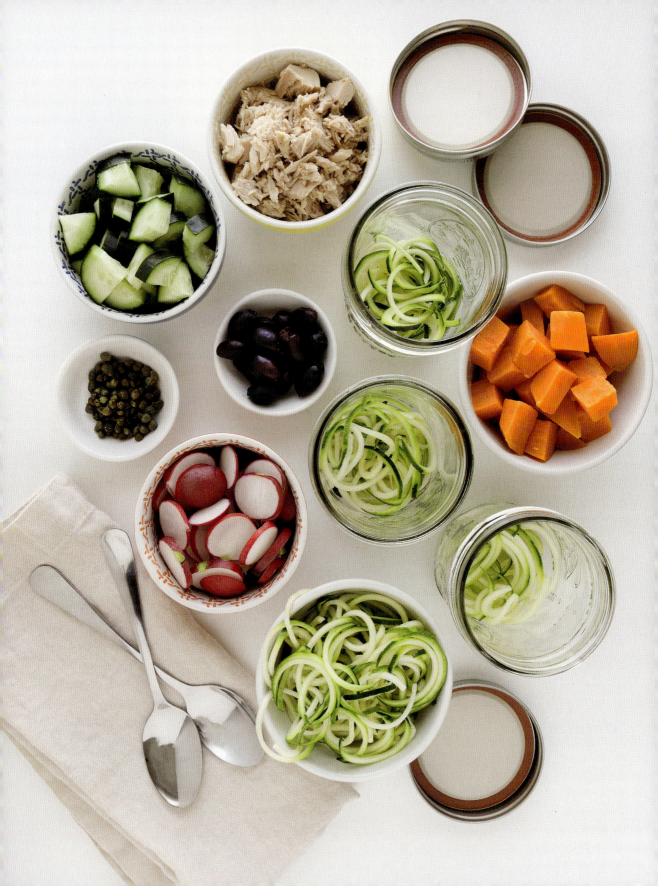

NIÇOISE SALAD

This egg-free Niçoise doesn't skimp on flavor—or on protein, fiber, and nutrients. For best results, store the dressing in a small portable container and add it just before you're ready to eat (this will prevent it from solidifying around the vegetables at the bottom). At mealtime, simply pour in the dressing, close the jar, and shake well, then enjoy the salad straight from the container or transfer to a bowl and dig in.

Prep time:
20 minutes
Cook time:
10 minutes
Yield:
4 servings

1 sweet potato, about 10 ounces (280 g)

1 zucchini, about ¾ pound (340 g)

1 cucumber, about ¾ pound (340 g)

8 radishes

2 (5-ounce [140 g]) cans tuna, drained

1 recipe Vinaigrette (page 185)

½ cup (55 g) sliced black olives

2 tablespoons (20 g) capers

1. Peel the sweet potato, then dice into ½-inch (1 cm) pieces. Place in a saucepan, cover with water, and bring to a boil over high heat. Reduce the heat to medium and cook, partially covered, until tender, about 10 minutes.

2. Meanwhile, cut off the top and bottom of the zucchini and spiralize with a vegetable spiralizer or peeler to make "noodles." Dice the cucumber and thinly slice the radishes. Break up large chunks of tuna with a fork if necessary.

3. Prepare the Vinaigrette following the directions on page 185.

To assemble: Divide the ingredients evenly among 4 glass jar containers, starting with the vinaigrette (unless you prefer to add the dressing later), followed by the zucchini noodles, cucumbers, tuna, sweet potatoes, radishes, olives, and capers.

Note: Store for up to 5 days in an airtight container in the refrigerator. Not suitable for freezing.

CARROT CAKE MUFFINS

If you're a fan of carrot cake, you'll love these little Carrot Cake Muffins. Thanks to aromatic spices like cinnamon, ginger, and cloves, they're bursting with the same wonderful flavor, but they're much healthier than the original version! Don't hesitate to double the ingredients during your batch-cooking session: These little gems freeze beautifully.

Prep time:
12 minutes
Cook time:
25 minutes
Yield:
5 servings

⅓ cup (40 g) cassava flour

⅓ cup (40 g) tigernut flour

2 tablespoons (16 g) coconut flour

½ teaspoon ground cinnamon

½ teaspoon ginger powder

¼ teaspoon baking powder (see page 29)

Pinch ground cloves

Pinch sea salt

¼ cup (60 g) palm shortening, melted

¼ cup (60 g) unsweetened applesauce

3 tablespoons (45 ml) maple syrup

½ tablespoon unflavored gelatin powder

½ cup (55 g) shredded carrot

1. Preheat the oven to 375°F (190°C or gas mark 5) and place the rack in the middle. Line a muffin pan with 5 greaseproof muffin liners.

2. In a large bowl, combine the three flours, cinnamon, ginger, baking powder, cloves, and salt.

3. In a small bowl, whisk together the palm shortening, applesauce, and maple syrup. Sprinkle the gelatin powder over the mixture, let it bloom for a couple of minutes, then whisk until well blended, ensuring there are no lumps. Mix in the shredded carrots.

4. Pour the liquid mixture over the dry ingredients and mix well with a spatula to obtain a smooth batter. Divide the batter evenly among the 5 muffin cups and press down lightly with your fingers. (This prevents air pockets from forming so that the dough holds together better once baked.)

5. Bake in the oven until the edges are lightly browned, about 25 minutes, or until a toothpick inserted near the center of a muffin comes out clean. Allow to cool completely on a cooling rack before storing.

Note: Store for up to 5 days in an airtight container, or freeze for up to 4 months.

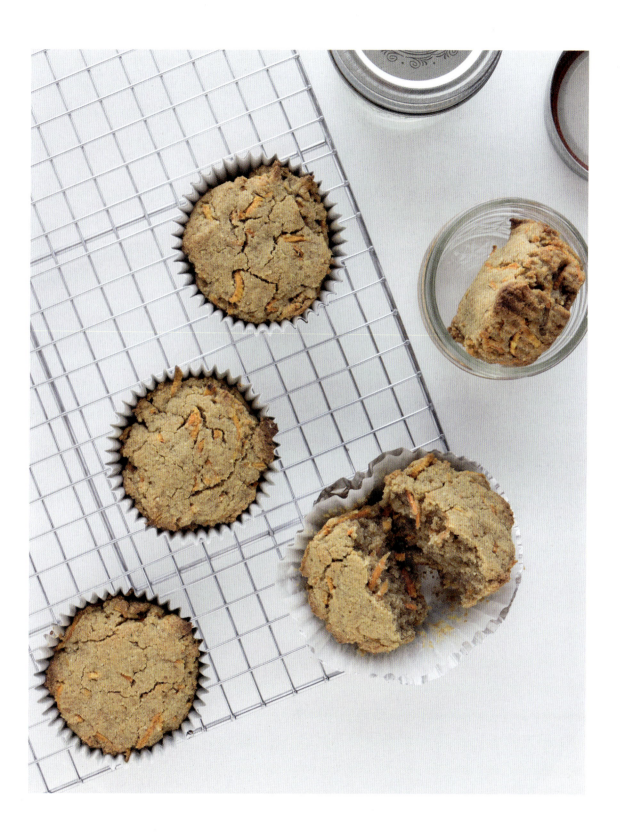

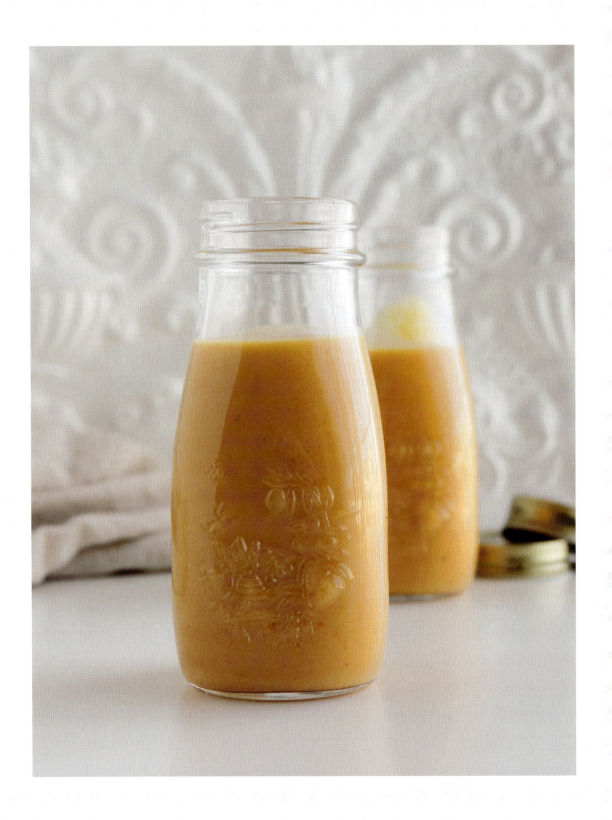

Chapter 5
EASY-PEASY MEAL PLAN

his simple, no-fuss meal plan may feature especially easy-to-follow directions and minimal cleanup, but that doesn't mean that your menu this week will be bland or boring! Just the opposite, in fact. The Easy-Peasy Meal Plan is big on flavor, so you can look forward to a healthy soup, creamy sauces, and a Sweet and Sour Asian Dressing you'll want to add to your list of favorites.

My **Sweet Potato Bisque**, creamy with just a hint of sweetness, is like a warm, fuzzy blanket for your belly. Add some protein, such as shredded chicken or cooked ground meat, to make it a full meal. The **Ginger Applesauce** is your snack this week, while the **Harvest Skillet**, packed with nourishing vegetables and tasty bacon, is easy to reheat for a quick and satisfying meal any time of the day. Skillet meals aren't just for breakfast anymore!

Then, the **Sweet and Sour Asian Cod with Rainbow Slaw** adds a whole bunch of colors to your plate thanks to a bright, showstopping slaw that's laced with a delightful sweet and sour dressing. But if it's more comfort food you're after, you'll fall in love with the **Chicken Marsala**. Served with Sweet Potato Mash and a creamy mushroom-based sauce, it's even better than the traditional version.

Kitchen note: Make sure you have 1 quart + 1½ cups (1 L + 355 ml) of chicken Bone Broth ready for your batch-cooking session.

	BREAKFAST	LUNCH	DINNER	SNACK
DAY 1	Harvest Skillet	Sweet Potato Bisque	Chicken Marsala	Ginger Applesauce
DAY 2	Chicken Marsala	Sweet and Sour Asian Cod	Harvest Skillet	Ginger Applesauce
DAY 3	Sweet Potato Bisque	Harvest Skillet	Sweet and Sour Asian Cod	Ginger Applesauce
DAY 4	Harvest Skillet	Sweet and Sour Asian Cod	Chicken Marsala	Ginger Applesauce
DAY 5	Sweet Potato Bisque	Chicken Marsala	Sweet and Sour Asian Cod	Ginger Applesauce

EXTRA SERVINGS: 2 Sweet Potato Bisque

Shopping List

PRODUCE

1 lime

3 scallions

4 cloves garlic

⅓ cup (80 ml) grape juice

4 radishes (4 ounces [112 g])

1 baby bok choy (5 ounces [168 g])

¼ purple cabbage (½ pound [227 g])

½ pound (227 g) mushrooms

¾ pound (340 g) broccoli florets

4 carrots (¾ pound [340 g])

2 onions (1 pound 1 ounce [476 g])

3 parsnips (1 pound 1 ounce [476 g])

2 pounds (908 g) orange sweet potatoes

2 pounds (908 g) white sweet potatoes

3 pounds (1362 g) apples + 2 apples (¾ pound [340 g])

MEAT/SEAFOOD

¾ pound (340 g) bacon

1¼ pounds (568 g) chicken breast tenders

4 (6-ounce [168 g]) cod fish fillets

1 quart + 1½ cups (1 L + 355 ml) chicken Bone Broth (page 180)

HERBS AND SPICES

¼ teaspoon garlic powder

1 teaspoon ginger powder

1 teaspoon dried parsley

1 tablespoon (2 g) dried sage

PANTRY ITEMS

2 teaspoons arrowroot flour

1 tablespoon (20 g) honey

2 tablespoons (30 ml) apple cider vinegar

2 tablespoons (30 ml) avocado oil

5 tablespoons (75 ml) coconut aminos

1¾ cups (415 ml) full-fat coconut milk

OTHER

Coconut oil

Extra-virgin olive oil

Sea salt

Equipment and Tools

15 containers for meals + 5 containers for snacks
    (see pages 32 to 33)

cutting board

immersion blender

large skillet (at least 11 inches [28 cm] wide)

measuring cups and spoons

paper towels

paring knife, serrated knife, chef's knife

potato masher

pots and pans

slotted spoon

vegetable peeler

wooden spoon

Batch-Cooking Directions

1. Reminder: *The morning before*, defrost the meat/fish, if frozen. Make sure you have 1 quart + 1½ cups (1 L + 355 ml) of chicken **Bone Broth** (page 180) on hand. Prepare your containers.

2. Start your batch-cooking session by completing steps 1 and 2 of the **Sweet Potato Bisque** (page 55) and set a timer for 20 minutes. While the soup is cooking, complete steps 1 and 2 of the **Ginger Applesauce** (page 56) and set a timer for 30 minutes.

3. Complete steps 3 and 4 of the **Sweet Potato Bisque** (page 55), then assemble. Complete steps 1 and 2 of the **Sweet Potato Mash** (page 184) using the white sweet potatoes. Set a timer for 20 minutes.

4. When the apples are done, complete step 3 of the **Ginger Applesauce** (page 56) and assemble.

5. When the sweet potatoes are done, complete step 3 of the **Sweet Potato Mash** (page 184) and set aside to cool.

6. Complete steps 1 through 3 of the **Harvest Skillet** (page 59). While you are waiting for step 3 to finish, prepare the **Sweet and Sour Asian Dressing** (step 3 of **Sweet and Sour Asian Cod**, page 60) and refrigerate. Assemble the skillet.

7. Complete steps 1 and 2 of the **Sweet and Sour Asian Cod** (page 60) and assemble.

8. Make the **Chicken Marsala** (page 63), steps 1 through 3, and assemble.

SWEET POTATO BISQUE

Sweet, creamy, and velvety, this comforting bisque always hits the spot! Enjoy it as is, or fancy it up with avocado pieces, crumbled bacon, cooked ground meat of your choice, or minced fresh herbs and scallions. For a lighter version, try replacing the sweet potatoes with butternut squash.

Prep time:
10 minutes
Cook time:
20 minutes
Yield:
5 servings

2 pounds (908 g) orange sweet potatoes

2 carrots (about 7 ounces [196 g])

1 parsnip (about 5 ounces [140 g])

1 onion (about 5 ounces [140 g])

1 quart + 1 cup (1 L + 235 ml) chicken Bone Broth (page 180)

¾ cup (180 ml) full-fat coconut milk

Sea salt to taste

1. Peel and chop the sweet potatoes, carrots, and parsnip. Chop the onion. Add the vegetables and the chicken broth to a stockpot.

2. Cover and bring to a boil over high heat, then reduce the heat to medium and cook until the vegetables are tender, about 20 minutes.

3. Remove from the heat and blend with an immersion blender until smooth.

4. Stir in the coconut milk and season to taste with salt.

   To assemble: Divide the soup evenly among 5 containers or glass jars.

   Note: Store for up to 5 days in an airtight container in the refrigerator, or freeze for up to 4 months.

GINGER APPLESAUCE

Feel free to use just about any apple variety in this flavorful, sugar-free applesauce, but remember that the cooking time may vary significantly from one variety to another. Apples with red or yellow skin tend to cook much faster than their green-skinned counterparts. Honeycrisp, Golden Delicious, Jonagold, and McIntosh are all easy to cook and always deliver a wonderfully sweet taste. No need to add sweeteners!

Prep time:
10 minutes
Cook time:
30 minutes
Yield:
5 servings

3 pounds (1362 g) apples

1¼ cups (295 ml) water

2 tablespoons (30 ml) apple cider vinegar

¼ teaspoon ginger powder, or more to taste

1. Core and chop the apples.

2. Add the apples, water, and vinegar to a pot. Cover and simmer over medium heat, stirring regularly, until the apples are soft and tender, about 30 minutes. Make sure the pot neither boils over nor runs dry. If needed, reduce the heat slightly or add water, ¼ cup (60 ml) at a time.

3. Allow the mixture to cool a bit before mashing the apples with a fork or a potato masher for a chunky applesauce. If you prefer your applesauce very smooth, run it through a food processor.

To assemble: Divide the applesauce evenly among 5 containers.

Note: Store for up to 5 days in an airtight container in the refrigerator, or freeze for up to 4 months.

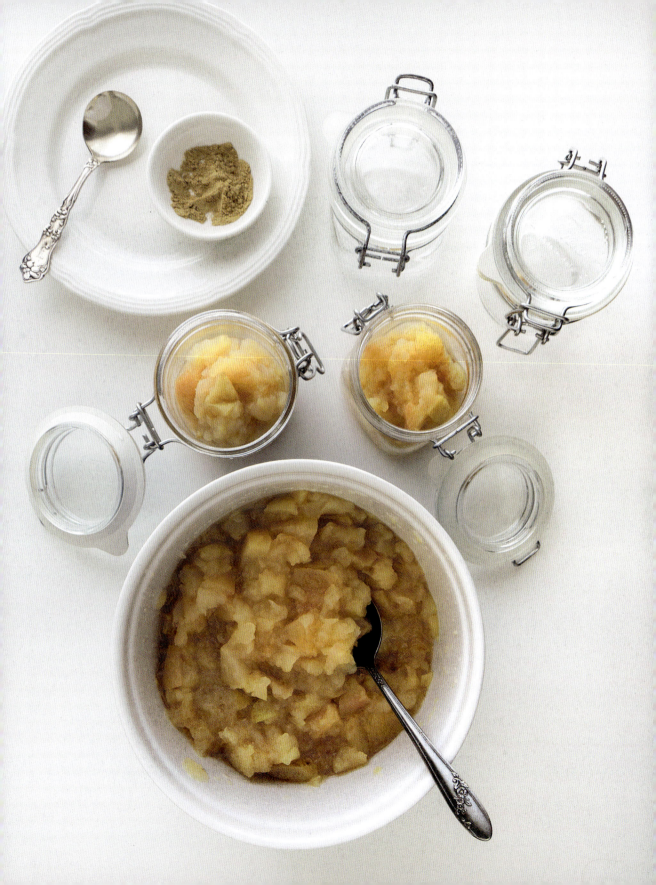

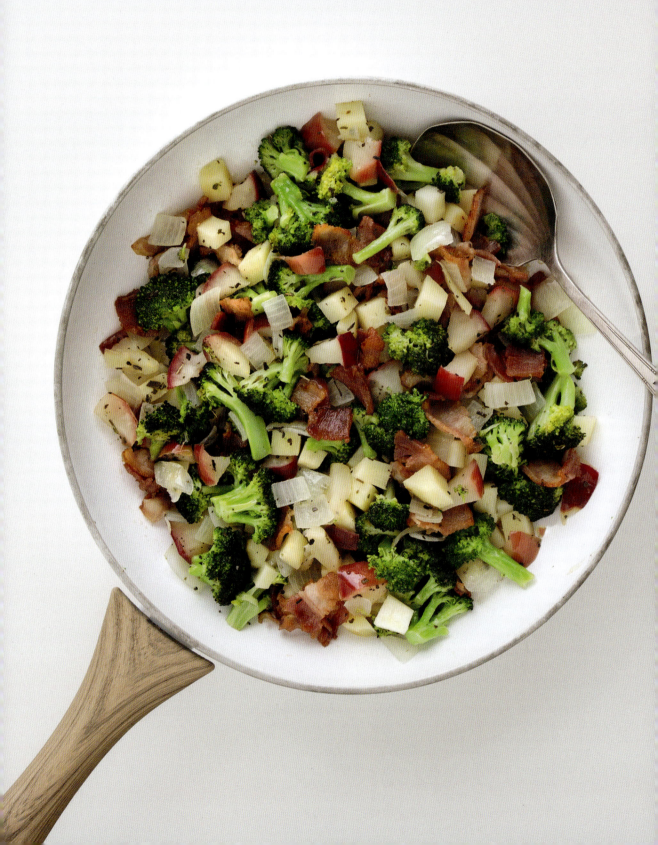

HARVEST SKILLET

Skillet meals rank high on my go-to recipes. This one-pan Harvest Skillet is easy to prepare, requires minimal cleanup, and always delivers a satisfying, highly nutritious meal. A word of advice: When you're buying bacon, carefully read the labels to avoid any ingredients on the Foods to Avoid list (page 18). Don't worry if you see cane sugar in the ingredients list, though: The sugar is "consumed" during the curing process.

Prep time:
10 minutes

Cook time:
24 minutes

Yield:
4 servings

¾ pound (340 g) bacon

¾ pound (340 g) broccoli florets

2 parsnips (about ¾ pound [340 g])

2 apples (about ¾ pound [340 g])

1 onion (about ¾ pound [340 g])

1 tablespoon (2 g) dried sage

½ teaspoon sea salt

1. Cut the bacon into 1-inch (2.5 cm) pieces. Add to a skillet and cook over medium heat for 12 minutes, or until golden, stirring a few times. When done, use a slotted spatula to transfer to a paper towel–lined plate, reserving the bacon fat in the skillet.

2. While the bacon is cooking, cut the broccoli florets into ½-inch (1 cm) pieces. Peel and dice the parsnips into ⅓-inch (8 mm) pieces. Core and chop the apples. Chop the onion.

3. Add the broccoli, parsnips, apples, onion, sage, and salt to the skillet. Cover and cook over medium heat, stirring a few times, until tender, about 12 minutes. Add the bacon back to the skillet and mix well. Check the seasoning and adjust to taste.

To assemble: Divide the mixture evenly among 4 containers.

Note: Store for up to 5 days in an airtight container in the refrigerator, or freeze for up to 4 months.

SWEET *and* SOUR ASIAN COD *with* RAINBOW SLAW

A mere 20 minutes is all it takes to whip up this healthy, colorful meal. Just be extra careful not to overcook the fish, especially if you are planning to reheat portioned meals later. If you do, the fish will turn hard and rubbery. Also, avoid reheating the cod in the microwave. Instead, warm it up slowly, covered, in a pan over low heat, and add some moisture such as oil or broth. Or you can skip the reheating altogether and enjoy it cold as a salad.

Prep time:
15 minutes
Cook time:
8 minutes
Yield:
4 servings

4 (6-ounce [168 g]) cod fish fillets

1 tablespoon (15 g) coconut oil

¼ teaspoon ginger powder

Sea salt to taste

FOR THE RAINBOW SLAW:

¼ purple cabbage (about ½ pound [227 g])

1 baby bok choy (about 5 ounces [140 g])

2 carrots (about 5 ounces [140 g])

4 radishes (about 4 ounces [112 g])

3 scallions

FOR THE SWEET AND SOUR ASIAN DRESSING:

3 tablespoons (45 ml) coconut aminos

2 tablespoons (30 ml) avocado oil

1 tablespoon (20 g) honey

Juice of 1 lime

½ teaspoon ginger powder

¼ teaspoon garlic powder

1. Pat the fish dry with paper towels. Melt the coconut oil in a large skillet over medium heat. Add the cod fillets, ginger powder, and salt to taste. Cover and cook for about 4 minutes on each side, until the fish is flaky. (Exact cooking time may vary according to the thickness of the fish.) Transfer to a plate to cool.

2. To prepare the slaw, thinly slice the cabbage, bok choy, carrots, radishes, and scallions. Place in a large bowl and mix well.

3. To prepare the dressing, combine the coconut aminos, avocado oil, honey, lime juice, ginger, and garlic powder in a bowl. Stir well and store in the refrigerator until needed.

To assemble: Divide the slaw evenly among 4 containers, then top each with a piece of cod. Reheat the fish separately and add the Asian dressing right before serving.

Note: Store for up to 5 days in an airtight container in the refrigerator. Not suitable for freezing.

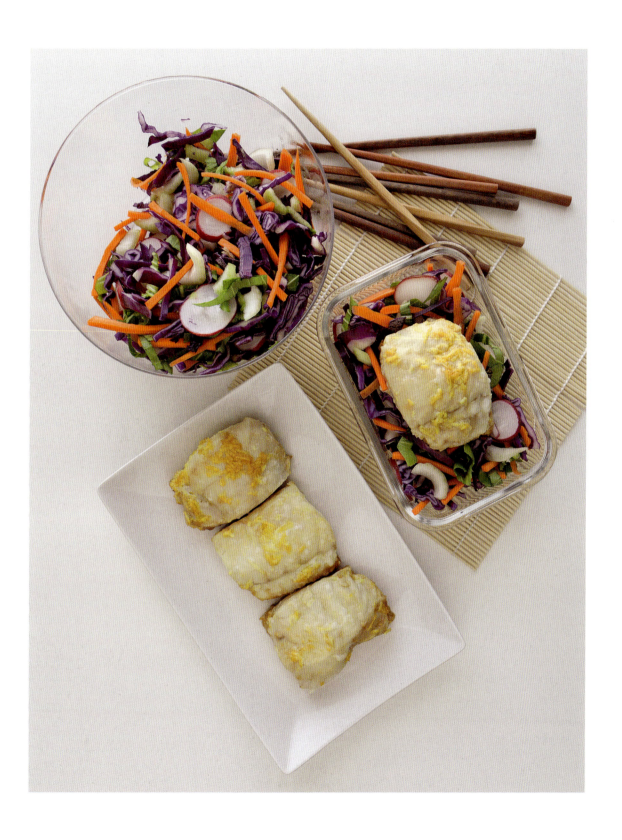

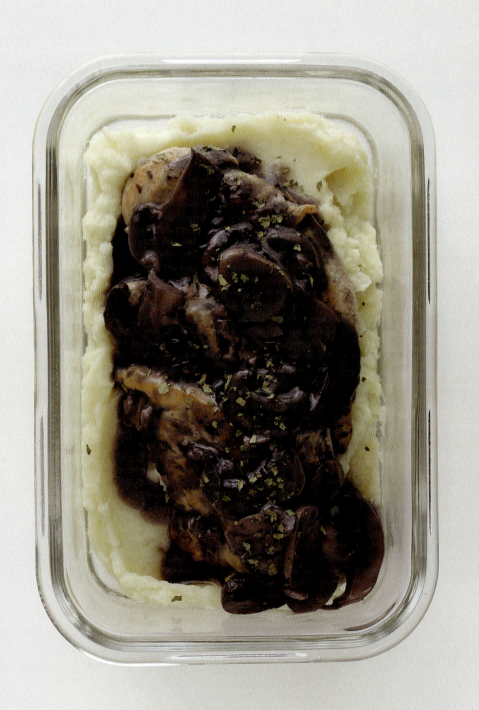

CHICKEN MARSALA *with* SWEET POTATO MASH

Here, the Marsala wine used in the original version of this dish is replaced with a combination of grape juice and liquid coconut aminos. Both lend flavor and richness to the sauce: You won't miss the Marsala a bit! This is a delicious, well-rounded meal with both sweet and earthy notes.

Prep time:
15 minutes
Cook time:
25 minutes
Yield:
4 servings

1¼ pounds (568 g) chicken breast tenders

Sea salt

1 tablespoon (15 ml) coconut oil, or more as needed

FOR THE MARSALA SAUCE:

½ pound (340 g) mushrooms

4 cloves garlic

2 tablespoons (30 ml) coconut oil

1 teaspoon dried parsley

2 tablespoons (20 ml) coconut aminos

½ cup (120 ml) chicken Bone Broth (page 180)

½ cup (120 ml) full-fat coconut milk

⅓ cup (80 ml) grape juice

½ teaspoon sea salt, or more to taste

2 teaspoons arrowroot flour

1 recipe white Sweet Potato Mash (page 184)

1. Pat the chicken breast tenders dry with a paper towel and season with salt on both sides. Heat the coconut oil in a large skillet over medium-high heat. When hot, add the chicken and cook until golden, about 2 minutes on each side. Transfer to a plate to cool. You may have to do this in two batches.

2. To make the sauce, thinly slice the mushrooms and mince the garlic. Melt the coconut oil in a clean large skillet over medium heat. When hot, add the mushrooms, garlic, parsley, and coconut aminos and cook, stirring frequently, for 5 minutes. Add the chicken broth, coconut milk, grape juice, and salt and continue to cook, covered, for an additional 10 minutes. Turn off the heat. Sprinkle the arrowroot flour over the mushroom sauce and stir well, making sure the flour is completely dissolved.

To assemble: Divide the ingredients evenly among 4 containers. Start with a layer of Sweet Potato Mash at the bottom, then top each with a quarter of the chicken and the Marsala sauce.

Note: Store for up to 5 days in an airtight container in the refrigerator, or freeze for up to 4 months.

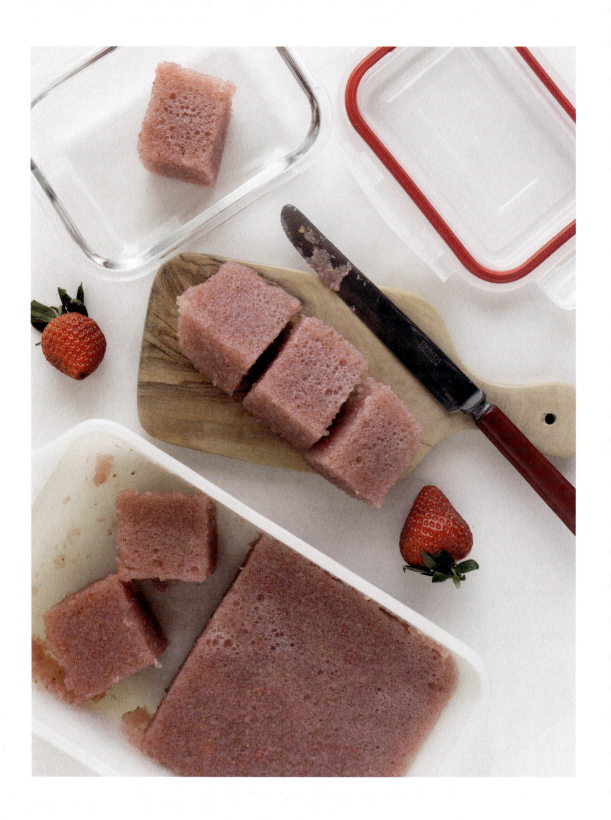

Chapter 6
LOW-FODMAP MEAL PLAN #1

S ome people will need to temporarily modify their AIP due to a FODMAP intolerance (that is, the malabsorption of fructose). FODMAP is an acronym for "fermentable, oligo-, di-, mono-saccharides, and polyols," a group of foods with a high content of short-chain carbohydrates that are rich in fructose. If you're sensitive to them, these foods can cause intestinal distress, such as bloating, gas, cramps, diarrhea, and constipation. But the good news is that following a low-FODMAP diet for a few weeks may have a dramatic effect on your symptoms.

This week's batch-cooking session begins with your snack! The **Strawberry Pâtes de Fruit** are super fun to eat; plus, they come with a secret gut-healing ingredient.

My colorful, festive **Baked Pesto Salmon** is served with Butternut Squash Rice, fresh young asparagus, and homemade Basil-Cilantro Pesto. The best part? You can make all this on a single sheet pan! Then there are the **Zucchini Boats with Marinara Sauce**, which are such a delicious way to add vegetables to your menu. The nightshade-free Marinara Sauce is a classic at my house, and it's a great partner for all kinds of meats and vegetables.

For something light and refreshing, you'll want to try the **Greek Salad with Tzatziki Dressing**. The star of the show is the herbed Tzatziki Dressing, of course: it's packed with cool cucumber, plus plenty of fresh dill and mint.

Finally, there's my **Morning Basil Skillet**, which isn't just for breakfast. A one-dish wonder, it's a simple yet elegant skillet meal featuring spinach, bok choy, and white sweet potatoes.

Kitchen note: If you feel hungry between meals, you can always supplement your menu with AIP- and low-FODMAP-approved snacks, such as fruit (strawberries, bananas, cantaloupe), olives, or baked sweet potatoes.

	BREAKFAST	LUNCH	DINNER	SNACK
DAY 1	Morning Basil Skillet	Greek Salad with Tzatziki Dressing	Zucchini Boats with Marinara Sauce	Strawberry Pâtes de Fruit
DAY 2	Zucchini Boats with Marinara Sauce	Baked Pesto Salmon	Greek Salad with Tzatziki Dressing	Strawberry Pâtes de Fruit
DAY 3	Morning Basil Skillet	Greek Salad with Tzatziki Dressing	Baked Pesto Salmon	Strawberry Pâtes de Fruit
DAY 4	Zucchini Boats with Marinara Sauce	Baked Pesto Salmon	Greek Salad with Tzatziki Dressing	Strawberry Pâtes de Fruit
DAY 5	Morning Basil Skillet	Zucchini Boats with Marinara Sauce	Baked Pesto Salmon	Strawberry Pâtes de Fruit

EXTRA SERVINGS: 1 Morning Basil Skillet

Shopping List

PRODUCE

4 cloves garlic

2 tablespoons (8 g) minced fresh dill

2 tablespoons (8 g) minced fresh mint

5 tablespoons (75 ml) lemon juice (from 2 lemons)

3 ounces (84 g) fresh basil

3 ounces (84 g) fresh cilantro

1 head butter lettuce

½ pound (227 g) beets

½ pound (227 g) carrots

1 sweet potato (½ pound [227 g])

1 English cucumber (¾ pound [340 g])

1 bunch young asparagus (1 pound [454 g])

2 bunches spinach (1 pound [454 g])

1 pound (454 g) strawberries

1 white sweet potato (1 pound [454 g])

3 baby bok choy (1¼ pounds [568 g])

1 butternut squash (2 pounds [908 g])

4 (8-ounce [227 g]) zucchini

MEAT/SEAFOOD

1⅓ cups (315 ml) chicken Bone Broth (page 180)

¾ pound (340 g) ground beef

1¼ pounds (568 g) boneless skinless chicken breasts

1½ pounds (680 g) ground pork

4 (6-ounce [168 g]) salmon fillets

HERBS AND SPICES

2 teaspoons dried marjoram

3½ teaspoons (2 g) dried basil

1 tablespoon (2 g) dried oregano

1 tablespoon (2 g) dried parsley

PANTRY ITEMS

1 tablespoon (8 g) arrowroot flour

1½ tablespoons (23 ml) maple syrup

2 tablespoons (30 ml) balsamic vinegar

3 tablespoons (24 g) gelatin powder

⅓ cup (32 g) kalamata olives

5 tablespoons (75 ml) coconut aminos

5 ounces (140 g) coconut milk yogurt

OTHER

Coconut oil

Extra-virgin olive oil

Sea salt

Equipment and Tools

15 containers for your meals + 5 containers for snacks (see pages 32 to 33)

9 x 5-inch (23 x 12.7 cm) glass baking dish

chef's knife

cutting board

food processor with S-blade

large rimmed baking sheet (12 x 17 inches [30.5 x 43 cm])

large skillet (at least 11 inches [28 cm] wide)

measuring cups and spoons

mixing bowls (small and large)

parchment paper

pots and pans

resealable plastic bag

slotted spatula

vegetable peeler

Batch-Cooking Directions

1. Reminder: *The morning before*, defrost the meat/seafood if frozen. *The day before*, make the **Greek Salad with Tzatziki Dressing** (page 74), steps 1 and 2. Make sure you have 1⅓ cups (315 ml) of chicken **Bone Broth** (page 180) on hand. Prepare your containers.

2. Start your batch-cooking session with the **Strawberry Pâtes de Fruit** (page 69), steps 1 through 5, and refrigerate.

3. Preheat the oven to 400°F (200°C or gas mark 6) and place the rack in the middle. Complete the **Baked Pesto Salmon** (page 70), steps 1 through 6, and assemble.

4. Make the **Zucchini Boats with Marinara Sauce** (page 73), steps 1 through 6, and assemble.

5. Complete the **Greek Salad with Tzatziki Dressing** (page 74), steps 3 through 5, and assemble.

6. Finish your batch-cooking session with the **Morning Basil Skillet** (page 77), steps 1 through 5, and assemble.

7. Don't forget to assemble the **Strawberry Pâtes de Fruit** (page 69) once the gelatin has set!

STRAWBERRY PÂTES *de* FRUIT

Unlike their traditional counterparts, these little pâtes de fruit are very low in sugar, but they're absolutely delicious: They taste a lot like a strawberry milk shake! Packed with fresh strawberries, rich in antioxidants, and gelatin powder, they're the best gut-healing treat around—and with only three ingredients (plus water), they couldn't be simpler to prepare.

Prep time:
8 minutes
Cook time:
3 minutes
Yield:
5 servings

1 pound (454 g) strawberries

1⅓ cups (315 ml) water, divided

3 tablespoons (28 g) gelatin powder

1½ tablespoons (23 ml) maple syrup, or more to taste

1. Lightly grease a 9 x 5-inch (23 x 12.7 cm) glass baking dish.

2. In a food processor equipped with an S-blade, add the strawberries and 1 cup (235 ml) of the water. Process until smooth, about 30 seconds.

3. In a small bowl, combine the remaining ⅓ cup (80 ml) water and gelatin powder. Mix well, making sure all the powder is dissolved and you obtain a gel-like mixture.

4. Transfer the strawberry mixture, gelatin, and maple syrup to a saucepan. Warm over medium-low heat for a few minutes, stirring constantly, until all the ingredients are well combined. Do not boil.

5. Pour the strawberry mixture into the dish and refrigerate for at least 4 hours, or until firm, preferably overnight.

To assemble: Cut the pâtes de fruit into small portions and divide evenly among 5 containers.

Note: Store for up to 7 days in an airtight container in the refrigerator. Not suitable for freezing.

BAKED PESTO SALMON

A layer of zippy Basil-Cilantro Pesto (page 178) really turns up the flavor on this easy sheet pan meal. When you're making the pesto, be sure to omit the garlic if you're following a low-FODMAP diet. And as a rule, it's best to add the pesto only during the last 5 minutes of cooking to maximize taste and nutrients. Of course, you can enjoy the pesto raw, too: Drizzle it on practically anything, especially roasted vegetables and meats.

Prep time:
15 minutes

Cook time:
25 minutes

Yield:
4 servings

1 butternut squash (2 pounds [908 g])

1 recipe Basil-Cilantro Pesto (page 178)

1 bunch young asparagus (1 pound [454 g])

2 tablespoons (30 ml) extra-virgin olive oil, divided, plus more for coating

¾ teaspoon sea salt, divided, plus more to taste

4 (6-ounce [168 g]) salmon fillets

1. Preheat the oven to 400°F (200°C or gas mark 6) and place the rack in the middle. Line a large rimmed baking sheet with parchment paper.

2. Cut off the top and bottom of the butternut squash. Peel and slice in half lengthwise. Scoop out and discard the seeds. Chop the flesh and rice it using a food processor equipped with an S-blade. You may have to do this in several batches. Transfer the "rice" to a bowl and rinse the food processor.

3. Prepare the Basil-Cilantro Pesto following the directions on page 178, omitting the garlic to make it low-FODMAP friendly.

4. Cut off 1 inch (2.5 cm) from the ends of the asparagus and discard. Combine the asparagus in a bowl with 1 tablespoon (15 ml) of the olive oil and ¼ teaspoon of the salt. Mix well and spread in a single layer on one side of the baking sheet. Place in the oven and roast for 10 minutes (set a timer).

5. Meanwhile, rub the salmon with oil and season with salt. When the timer goes off, place the salmon on the other half of the baking sheet and continue to roast for 5 minutes (set a timer again). When the timer goes off, coat the salmon to taste with pesto and roast for another 5 minutes.

6. Heat the remaining 1 tablespoon (15 ml) olive oil in a large skillet over medium heat. When hot, add the butternut squash "rice" and remaining ½ teaspoon salt. Mix well and cook until crisp-tender, about 5 minutes. Don't overcook the "rice" or it will turn mushy.

To assemble: Divide the ingredients evenly among 4 containers, starting with a layer of butternut squash rice at the bottom, followed by the salmon and asparagus.

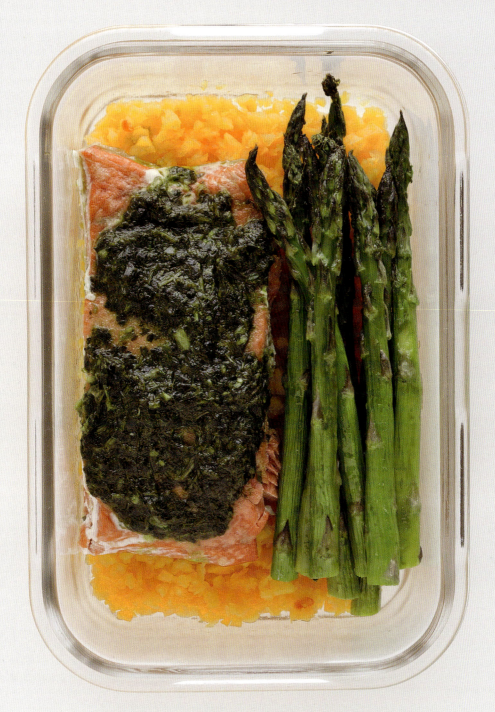

Note: Store for up to 5 days in an airtight container in the refrigerator, or freeze for up to 4 months.

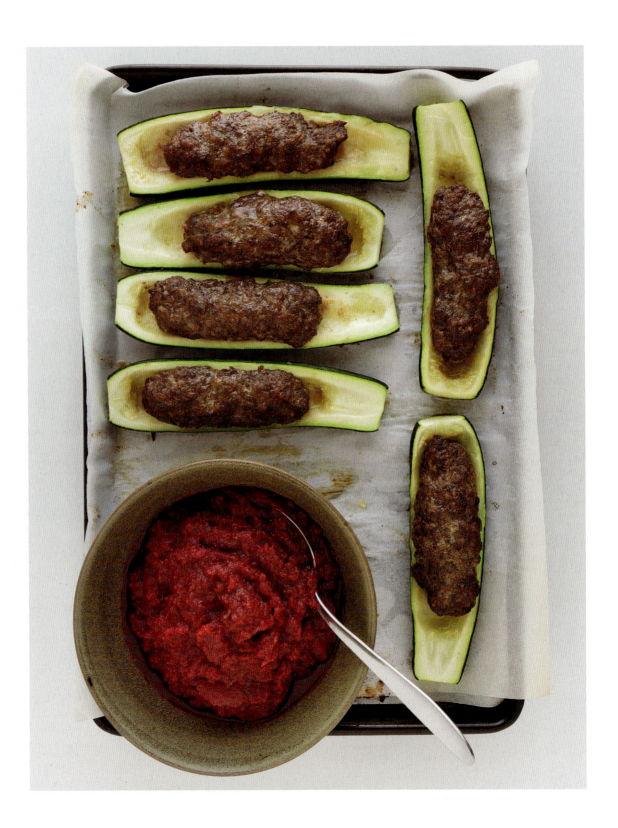

ZUCCHINI BOATS *with* MARINARA SAUCE

Stuffed vegetables are an easy way to add a substantial amount of fiber to your diet, and they're always fun to eat. (Your kids are sure to agree!) I use zucchini in this recipe, but feel free to experiment with other stuffable vegetables, like tomatoes and bell peppers (after the reintroduction phase, that is).

Prep time:
20 minutes
Cook time:
40 minutes
Yield:
4 servings

1 recipe Marinara Sauce (page 183)

4 (8-ounce [227 g]) zucchini

¾ pound (340 g) ground beef

½ pound (227 g) ground pork

2 tablespoons (30 ml) coconut aminos

1 tablespoon (8 g) arrowroot flour

1 tablespoon (2 g) dried parsley

1 teaspoon sea salt, plus more for sprinkling

1. Preheat the oven to 400°F (200°C or gas mark 6) and place the rack in the middle. Line a rimmed baking sheet with parchment paper.

2. Start cooking the vegetables for the Marinara Sauce, following the directions on page 183, step 1. Set a timer for 30 minutes.

3. While the vegetables for the sauce are boiling, cut off and discard the tops and bottoms of the zucchini, then slice the zucchini in half lengthwise. Scoop out and discard the seedy core. Sprinkle the inside of the zucchini with salt.

4. Combine the ground beef, ground pork, coconut aminos, arrowroot flour, parsley, and salt in a bowl. Mix thoroughly using your hands and divide into 8 equal portions.

5. Stuff each zucchini half with one portion of meat, then line up the prepared zucchini on the baking sheet. Bake in the oven until the meat is no longer pink inside and the zucchini is tender, about 25 minutes.

6. When the timer goes off for the boiling vegetables, finish preparing the Marina Sauce.

To assemble: Divide the ingredients evenly among 4 containers, placing the zucchini boats at the bottom before coating them with a serving of Marinara Sauce.

Note: Store for up to 5 days in an airtight container in the refrigerator, or freeze for up to 4 months.

GREEK SALAD *with* TZATZIKI DRESSING

Guidelines issued by Monash University, the home of a world-renowned research team studying the low-FODMAP diet, recommend keeping your consumption of canned coconut milk to a maximum of ½ cup (120 ml) per day if you have sorbitol malabsorption. And if you know coconut milk is a trigger for you, skip the tzatziki dressing altogether and replace it with plain chopped cucumber plus some Mayonnaise (page 181). To make this salad more filling, add a serving of Cauliflower Rice (page 177).

Prep time:
15 minutes
Cook time:
15 minutes
Yield:
4 servings

1¼ pounds (568 g) boneless skinless chicken breasts

⅓ cup (32 g) kalamata olives

FOR THE MARINADE:

¼ cup (60 ml) extra-virgin olive oil

3 tablespoons (45 ml) lemon juice

½ tablespoon dried basil

½ tablespoon dried oregano

1 teaspoon sea salt

4 zucchini (1¼ pounds [568 g]), chopped

1 recipe Tzatziki Dressing (page 186)

1 head butter lettuce

1. Cut the chicken breasts into bite-size pieces and place in a large resealable plastic bag. Crush the olives with the flat side of a chef's knife and add to the bag as well.

2. To make the marinade, in a bowl, combine the olive oil, lemon juice, basil, oregano, and salt. Stir well, then pour over the chicken. Seal the bag and massage the marinade into the chicken, making sure all the pieces are well coated. Place in the refrigerator overnight (or for at least 2 hours), turning the bag over a few times.

3. Heat a large skillet over medium heat. When hot, add the chicken (including the leftover marinade) and cook, covered, until no longer pink inside, about 8 minutes. Transfer to a plate with a slotted spatula and return the skillet to the heat (including the cooking juices).

4. Increase the heat to medium-high, add the zucchini, and cook until crisp-tender, about 6 minutes.

5. Prepare the Tzatziki Dressing following the directions on page 186. Core the butter lettuce and separate the leaves.

To assemble: Divide the ingredients evenly among 4 containers, starting with the lettuce leaves at the bottom, followed by the chicken and zucchini. Top each with a dollop of Tzatziki Dressing. Alternatively, you can store this salad in a glass jar, starting with the meat at the bottom, followed by the zucchini, Tzatziki Dressing, and finally the lettuce.

Note: Store for up to 5 days in an airtight container in the refrigerator. Not suitable for freezing.

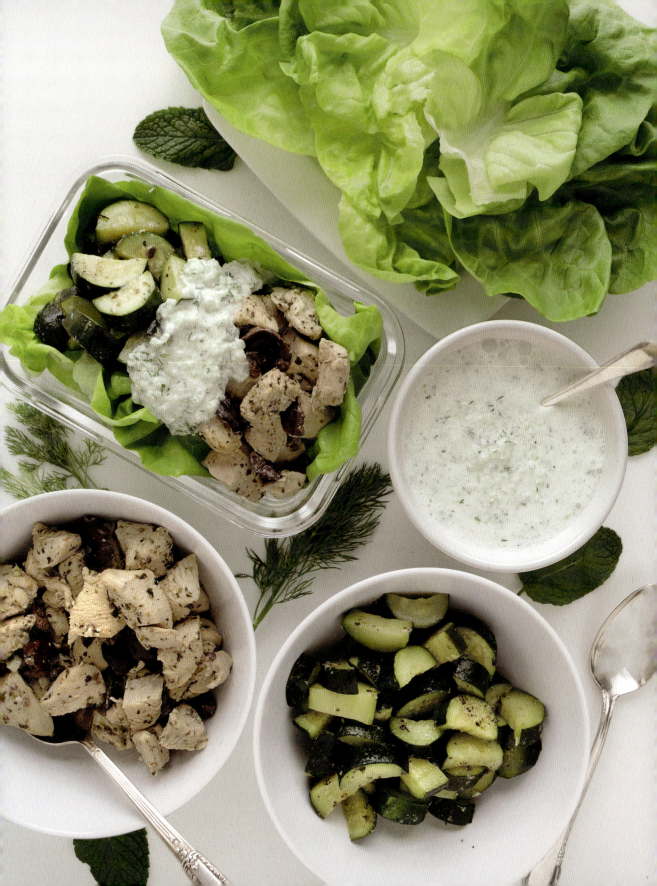

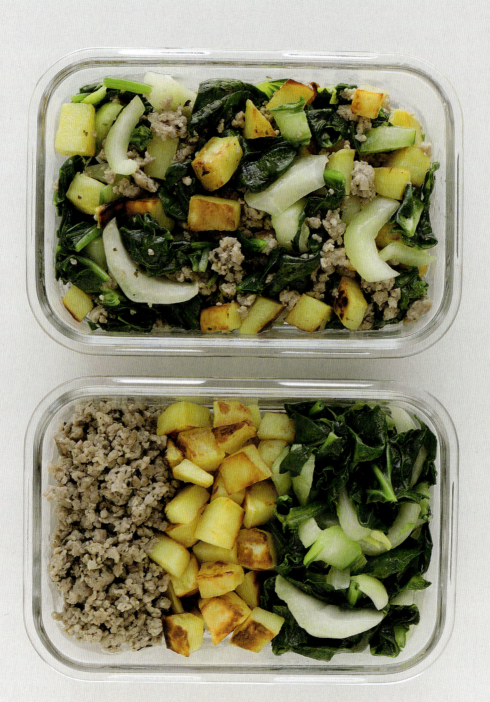

MORNING BASIL SKILLET

Skillets make it easy to create balanced meals with proteins, vegetables, and healthy fats. They're quick to throw together, and because they're prepared in a single skillet or frying pan, cleanup is a breeze! This version, which is packed with bok choy, spinach, and white sweet potatoes, offers an ideal combination of high- and low-starch vegetables for a nutritious meal that'll give you hours of energy.

Prep time:
10 minutes
Cook time:
25 minutes
Yield:
4 servings

3 baby bok choy (1¼ pounds [568 g])

2 bunches spinach (1 pound [454 g])

1 white sweet potato (1 pound [454 g])

3 tablespoons (45 ml) extra-virgin olive oil, divided

1¾ teaspoons sea salt, divided

1 pound (454 g) ground pork

1 teaspoon dried basil

1 tablespoon (15 ml) coconut oil

1. Slice the bok choy and spinach. Peel and dice the sweet potato into ⅓-inch (8 mm) pieces, place in a bowl, and cover with water (to prevent oxidation).

2. Heat 1 tablespoon (15 ml) of the olive oil in a large skillet over medium heat. When hot, add the bok choy and ¼ teaspoon of the salt and cook until crisp-tender, about 6 minutes. Transfer to a plate, then return the skillet to the heat.

3. Heat another 1 tablespoon (15 ml) of the olive oil in the skillet. When hot, add the spinach and ¼ teaspoon of the salt and cook until wilted, 2 to 3 minutes. Transfer to a plate, then return the skillet to the heat. You may have to do this in two batches.

4. Heat the remaining 1 tablespoon (15 ml) olive oil in the skillet. When hot, add the ground pork, ¾ teaspoon of the salt, and the dried basil. Mix well and cook until no longer pink, 5 to 6 minutes. Transfer to a plate with a slotted spatula and discard the cooking juices. Wipe the skillet clean.

5. Drain the sweet potatoes and pat dry with a paper towel. Heat the coconut oil over medium-high heat in the skillet. When hot, add the sweet potatoes and remaining ½ teaspoon salt and cook, turning them a few times, until cooked through and lightly golden, about 8 minutes.

To assemble: Divide the ingredients evenly among 4 containers. You may decide to keep the ingredients separated or mix them together, skillet style. Your choice.

Note: Store for up to 5 days in an airtight container in the refrigerator, or freeze for up to 4 months.

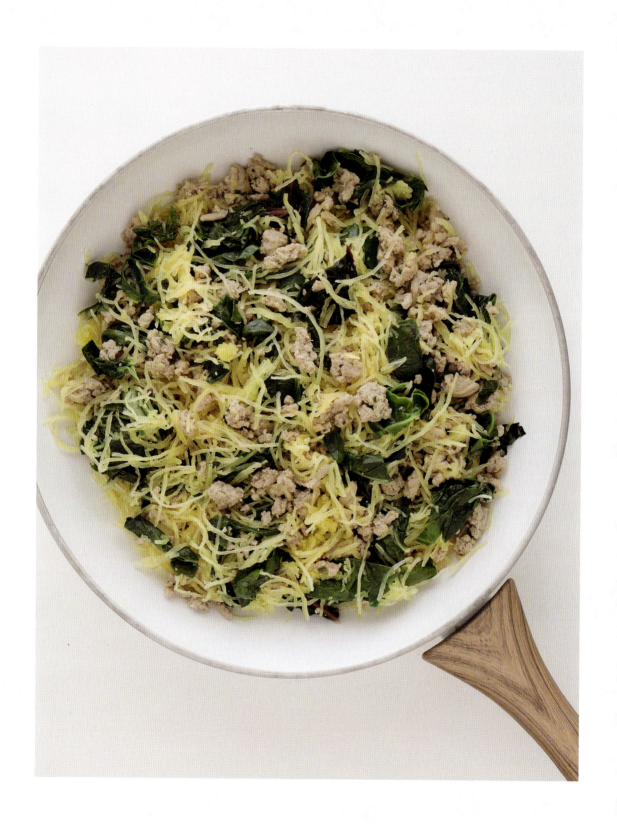

Chapter 7
LOW-FODMAP MEAL PLAN #2

You may be following a low-FODMAP menu this week, but that doesn't mean you'll feel deprived! Quite the opposite. The creative recipes in this menu draw on multiple sources of protein (meat, poultry, fish, and shellfish) and a wide variety of vegetables so that you'll always have delicious and satiating meals to look forward to.

Because all of these recipes are both AIP and low-FODMAP friendly, you can go ahead and enjoy them without worrying about triggering your symptoms. First up is the **Tarragon Turkey Skillet**, a perfect example of a quick and highly nutritious AIP meal, featuring a generous portion of Baked Spaghetti Squash, chard, and some easy-to-digest proteins.

You'll have fun preparing the **Salmon en Papillote**—that's a fancy French name describing a simple cooking technique, which consists of wrapping your food in parchment paper so that it steams in the oven, preserving the precious juices (and flavor!) of your ingredients.

The **Turmeric Squash Risotto with Ground Beef and Collard Greens** is another nutritional powerhouse, combining the anti-inflammatory benefits of ground turmeric and the antioxidants in bright-orange butternut squash (it's high in vitamin A and C). Next, to satisfy your craving for Asian food, comes the exotic, ultra-healthy **Shrimp Pad Thai**. It's served with zucchini noodles and julienned carrots, and just wait until you taste the sauce! (If you can't do shellfish, see the recipe headnote on page 88 to learn how to substitute with chicken.)

Your snack this week is simple and low-key: **Mixed Berries with Coconut Cream** are healthy and refreshing (and their bright, cheerful colors always put me in a good mood!).

Kitchen note: Make sure you have 1 cup (235 ml) of chicken Bone Broth available when you start the batch-cooking session.

	BREAKFAST	LUNCH	DINNER	SNACK
DAY 1	Tarragon Turkey Skillet	Shrimp Pad Thai	Salmon en Papillote	Mixed Berries with Coconut Cream
DAY 2	Turmeric Squash Risotto	Shrimp Pad Thai	Tarragon Turkey Skillet	Mixed Berries with Coconut Cream
DAY 3	Salmon en Papillote	Tarragon Turkey Skillet	Turmeric Squash Risotto	Mixed Berries with Coconut Cream
DAY 4	Tarragon Turkey Skillet	Salmon en Papillote	Shrimp Pad Thai	Mixed Berries with Coconut Cream
DAY 5	Turmeric Squash Risotto	Shrimp Pad Thai	Salmon en Papillote	Mixed Berries with Coconut Cream

EXTRA SERVINGS: 1 Turmeric Squash Risotto

Shopping List

PRODUCE

Handful of fresh cilantro

1 (½-inch [1 cm]) knob fresh ginger

4 limes (3 for juicing)

5 ounces (140 g) baby spinach

½ pound (227 g) carrots

¾ pound (340 g) blueberries

¾ pound (340 g) raspberries

1 bunch collard greens (¾ pound [340 g])

1 pound (454 g) strawberries

1 pound (454 g) summer yellow squash

2 bunches chard (½ to ¾ pound [227 to 340 g] each)

1 butternut squash (2 pounds [908 g])

1 spaghetti squash (3 pounds [1362 g])

3 pounds (1362 g) zucchini (about 3 medium zucchini)

MEAT/SEAFOOD

1 cup (235 ml) chicken Bone Broth (page 180)

1 pound (454 g) ground beef

1 pound (454 g) ground turkey

24 peeled, deveined shrimp (1 pound [454 g])

4 (6-ounce [168 g]) salmon fillets

HERBS AND SPICES

¾ teaspoon dried dill

1 teaspoon dried tarragon

1 teaspoon ground turmeric

OTHER

Coconut oil

Extra-virgin olive oil

Sea salt

PANTRY ITEMS

1 (14-ounce [392 ml]) can full-fat coconut milk

5 tablespoons (75 ml) maple syrup

2 tablespoons (30 ml) coconut aminos

2 tablespoons (30 ml) fish sauce

Equipment and Tools

15 containers for your meals + 5 containers for snacks (see pages 32 to 33)

baking dish

chef's knife

cutting board

food processor with S-blade

large rimmed baking sheet (12 x 17 [30.5 x 43 cm])

large skillet (at least 11 inches [28 cm] wide)

measuring cups and spoons

mixing bowls

parchment paper

slotted spatula

vegetable spiralizer

Batch-Cooking Directions

1. Reminder: *The morning before*, defrost the meat and fish if frozen. Make sure you have 1 cup (240 ml) of chicken **Bone Broth** (page 180) on hand. Prepare your containers.

2. Preheat the oven to 400°F (200°C or gas mark 6) and place the rack in the middle. Start your batch-cooking session with the **Tarragon Turkey Skillet** (page 83), step 1. Set a timer for 30 minutes.

3. While the spaghetti squash is cooking, complete steps 1 through 5 of the **Salmon en Papillote** (page 84).

4. When the timer goes off for the spaghetti squash, transfer it to a plate to cool. Put the **Salmon en Papillote** (page 84) in the oven and bake, following step 6. Set a timer for 15 minutes. Meanwhile, use a fork to scrape out the noodles from the spaghetti squash and set aside. Also, complete step 2 of the **Tarragon Turkey Skillet** (page 83).

5. When the timer goes off for the **Salmon en Papillote** (page 84), transfer the contents of the parchment paper packets to your containers.

6. Complete steps 3 through 5 of the **Tarragon Turkey Skillet** (page 83) and assemble.

7. Make the **Turmeric Squash Risotto** (page 87), steps 1 through 5, and assemble.

8. Make the **Shrimp Pad Thai** (page 88), steps 1 through 4, and assemble.

9. Make the **Mixed Berries with Coconut Cream** (page 91), step 1, and assemble.

TARRAGON TURKEY SKILLET *with* CHARD *and* SPAGHETTI SQUASH

By now you've probably noticed that I love skillet meals: They're such a handy way to make healthy meals with minimal fuss. In this one, spaghetti squash is the star of the show, and rightly so. Because it yields spaghetti-like strands when cooked, it's the ideal replacement for pasta, and it pairs well with almost any other ingredient. Feel free to swap turkey for any other ground meat of your choice, or replace the chard with kale or collard greens.

Prep time:
10 minutes
Cook time:
30 minutes
Yield:
4 servings

1 spaghetti squash (about 3 pounds [1362 g])

2 bunches chard (½ to ¾ pound [227 to 340 g] each)

2 tablespoons (30 ml) olive oil, divided

1 pound (454 g) ground turkey

¾ teaspoon sea salt

1 teaspoon dried tarragon

1. To prepare the Baked Spaghetti Squash, follow the oven directions on page 179.

2. While the spaghetti squash is cooking, remove the hard stems from the chard leaves, discard the stems, and chop the leaves.

3. Heat 1 tablespoon (15 ml) of the olive oil in a large skillet over medium heat. Add the chard and cook, covered, until wilted, about 2 minutes. You might have to do this in two batches. Transfer to a plate and set aside.

4. In the same skillet, heat the remaining 1 tablespoon (15 ml) olive oil. When hot, add the ground turkey, salt, and tarragon. Cook, uncovered, stirring frequently, until the meat is cooked through and no longer pink, about 6 minutes.

5. If desired, combine the spaghetti squash noodles, chard, and turkey in a large bowl. Mix well.

To assemble: Divide evenly among 4 containers. You may decide to keep the ingredients separated or mix them together, skillet style.

Note: Store for up to 5 days in an airtight container in the refrigerator, or freeze for up to 4 months.

SALMON EN PAPILLOTE

Papillote might sound like a complicated process, but it's actually very simple: It's just a French word describing food that's been steamed in the oven in tightly wrapped packets made of parchment paper. This way you preserve the food's moisture, texture, and flavor. I use salmon here, perched on a colorful layer of squash, zucchini, and spinach, but you can swap salmon for any other fish of your choice, like cod or halibut. Reheat slowly in a skillet over low heat, and add a drizzle of olive oil.

Prep time:
15 minutes
Cook time:
15 minutes
Yield:
4 servings

1 pound (454 g) yellow summer squash

1 pound (454 g) zucchini

5 ounces (140 g) baby spinach

4 (6-ounce [168 g]) salmon fillets (no thicker than 1 inch [2.5 cm])

4 tablespoons (60 ml) olive oil

¾ teaspoon dried dill

¾ teaspoon sea salt

1. Preheat the oven to 400°F (200°C or gas mark 6) and place the rack in the middle.

2. Cut off the tops and bottoms of the squash and zucchini, then dice and combine.

3. Cut four 15 x 15-inch (38 x 38 cm) pieces of parchment paper and lay them flat on your workspace.

4. Divide the squash mixture and spinach into 4 portions. Lay one portion of spinach and one portion of the squash mixture in the center of each piece of parchment paper, starting with the spinach at the bottom. Top each with a piece of salmon, then drizzle each with 1 tablespoon (15 ml) of olive oil and season with the dill and salt.

5. Bring two sides of the parchment paper together and fold several times. Repeat for the left and right sides, sealing the packet tightly. Don't worry if you didn't do this perfectly: The important thing is to make sure that the little packets are tightly sealed to prevent the steam from escaping during cooking.

6. Place the packets on a baking sheet. Bake for 15 minutes. You may have to adjust the cooking time according to the thickness of the fish. It's okay to open the packets to check for doneness (be careful—escaping steam will be hot), then reseal and continue to cook if needed.

To assemble: Transfer the contents of each packet to a container. Don't forget to drizzle the cooking juices on top!

Note: Store for up to 5 days in an airtight container in the refrigerator, or freeze for up to 4 months.

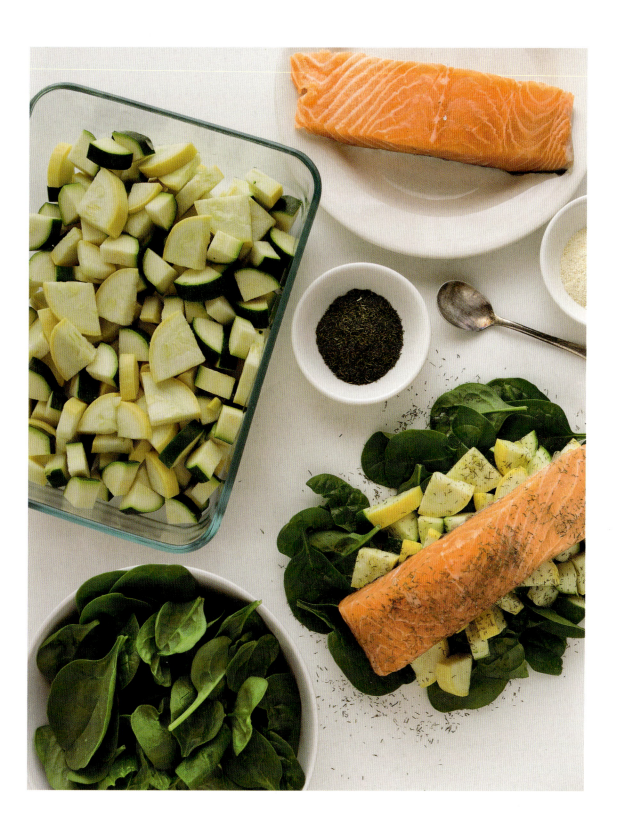

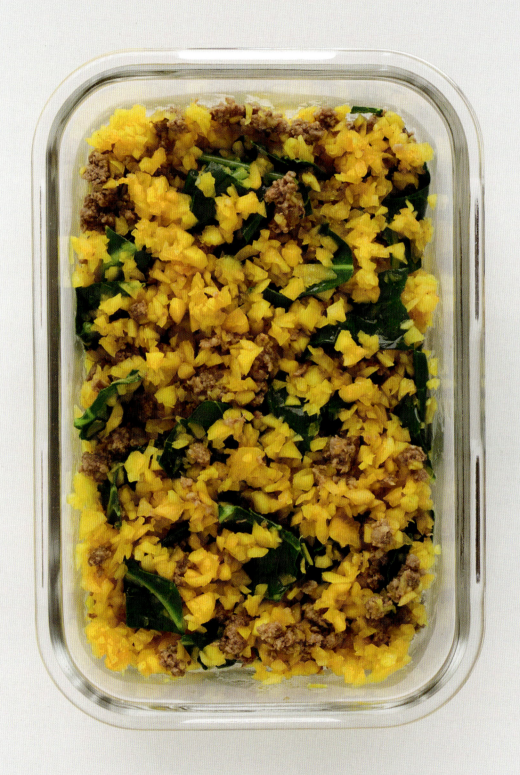

TURMERIC SQUASH RISOTTO *with* GROUND BEEF *and* COLLARD GREENS

Ah, turmeric, the golden hero of the AIP kitchen! Actually, it's turmeric's most active compound, curcumin, that deserves all the glory. This amazing spice is packed with health benefits: It's a potent anti-inflammatory and antioxidant and may have cancer-fighting properties, too. Pro tip: Combine turmeric with healthy fats to enhance its absorption. Oh, and feel free to add more than the suggested teaspoon in this recipe; more is better here!

Prep time:
15 minutes
Cook time:
20 minutes
Yield:
4 servings

1 butternut squash (2 pounds [908 g])

1 bunch collard greens (¾ pound [340 g])

2 tablespoons (30 ml) coconut oil, divided

1 pound (454 g) ground beef

1¾ teaspoons sea salt, divided

1 teaspoon ground turmeric

1 cup (240 ml) chicken Bone Broth (page 180)

1. Cut off the top and bottom of the butternut squash and discard. Peel and slice in half lengthwise. Scoop out and discard the seeds. Chop the flesh and rice it, using a food processor equipped with an S-blade. You may have to do this in several batches.

2. Remove and discard the hard stems from the collard greens, then chop the leaves.

3. Heat ½ tablespoon (8 ml) of the coconut oil in a large skillet over medium heat. When hot, add the ground beef and ¾ teaspoon of the salt, and cook until no longer pink, 7 to 8 minutes. Transfer to a large mixing bowl with a slotted spatula and wipe the skillet clean.

4. Add 1 tablespoon (15 ml) of the coconut oil, riced butternut squash, turmeric, remaining 1 teaspoon salt, and broth. Cover and cook until tender, about 5 minutes. Don't overcook the "rice" or it will become mushy.

5. Transfer the cooked "rice" to the mixing bowl. Wipe the skillet clean again and melt the remaining ½ tablespoon (8 ml) coconut oil. Add the collard greens and sauté until wilted, about 3 minutes. Transfer to the mixing bowl and mix well. Check the seasoning and adjust salt to taste.

To assemble: Divide the ingredients evenly among 4 containers.

Note: Store for up to 5 days in an airtight container in the refrigerator, or freeze for up to 4 months.

SHRIMP PAD THAI

If you've been craving Asian takeout, this Shrimp Pad Thai will do the trick! The sauce tastes amazing even on its own: It's the perfect blend of sweet and sour. This recipe calls for a lot of zucchini noodles, but don't be alarmed by the volume: The noodles reduce quite a bit during cooking. Prefer turf to surf? No problem—just swap the shrimp for diced chicken.

Prep time:
20 minutes
Cook time:
16 minutes
Yield:
4 servings

2 pounds (908 g) zucchini

½ pound (227 g) carrots

Juice of 3 limes

3 tablespoons (45 ml) maple syrup

2 tablespoons (30 ml) coconut aminos

2 tablespoons (30 ml) fish sauce

1 (½-inch [1.3 cm]) knob fresh ginger, peeled and grated

1 tablespoon (15 ml) coconut oil

24 peeled, deveined shrimp (about 1 pound [454 g])

¼ teaspoon sea salt

1 lime, cut into wedges, for garnish

Handful of cilantro, minced, for garnish

1. Cut off the tops and bottoms of the zucchini and discard. Spiralize the zucchini with a vegetable spiralizer to obtain "noodles." Peel and julienne the carrots. Set aside.

2. To prepare the sauce, combine the lime juice, maple syrup, coconut aminos, fish sauce, and grated ginger in a small bowl. Set aside.

3. Heat the coconut oil in a large skillet over medium heat. When hot, add the shrimp, and ¼ cup (60 ml) of the sauce, and sprinkle with salt. Toss and cook for 2 to 3 minutes on each side, until the shrimp turn pink and are cooked through. Transfer to a plate with a slotted spatula and set aside.

4. Add the rest of the sauce to the skillet, plus the carrots. Cook for 5 minutes. Add the zucchini and continue to cook, stirring occasionally, for an additional 5 minutes. (I prefer my pad Thai to be on the crisp-tender side; you have the option to let the vegetables cook longer if you prefer them fully cooked.)

To assemble: Divide the zucchini and carrot mixture evenly among 4 containers, top each with 6 shrimp, and drizzle with leftover sauce. Garnish with lime wedges and minced cilantro.

Note: Store for up to 5 days in an airtight container in the refrigerator. Not suitable for freezing.

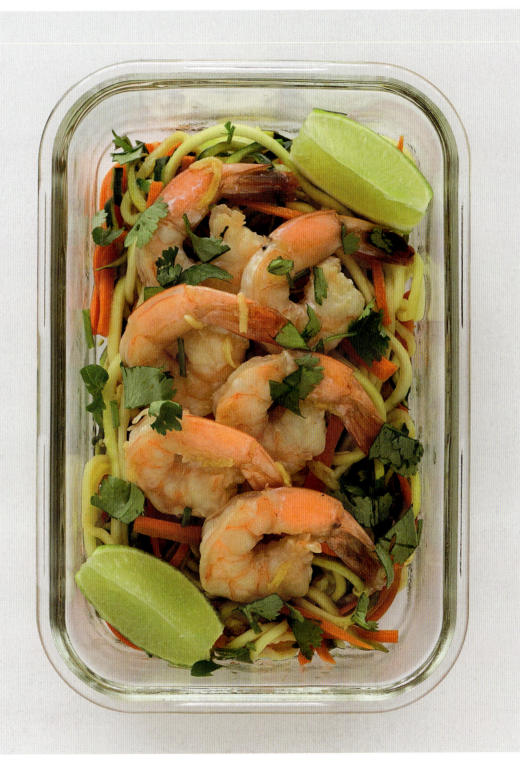

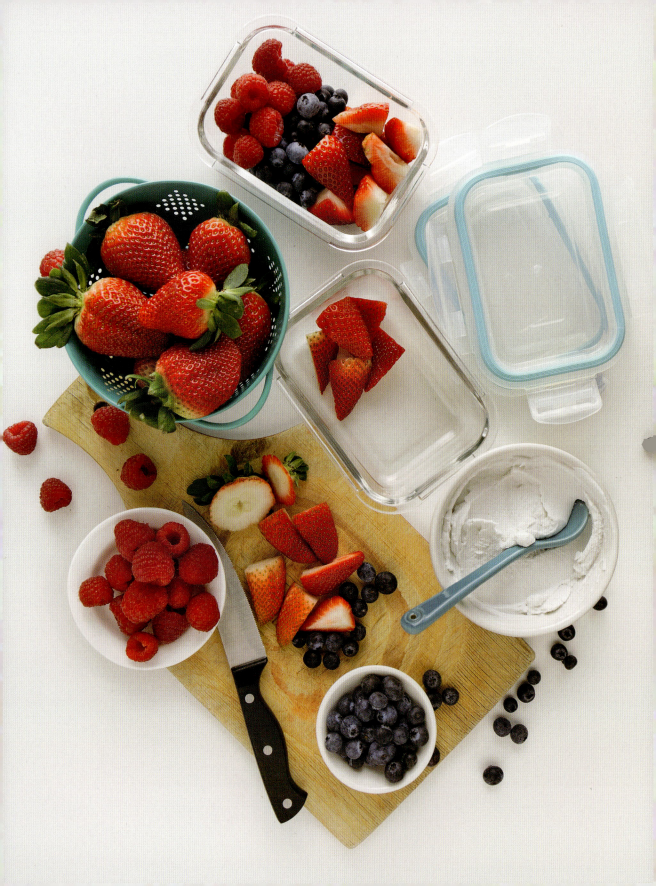

MIXED BERRIES *with* COCONUT CREAM

Fresh fruit, especially berries, is always a good choice for a quick-prep snack. Berries are full of antioxidants, and they contain less fructose than other fruits, like grapes and bananas. For a little indulgence, add some sweetened coconut cream—just keep your serving of coconut milk (or coconut cream) to a maximum of ½ cup (120 ml) per day if you have sorbitol malabsorption.

Prep time:
10 minutes
Cook time:
N/A
Yield:
5 servings

1 (14-ounce [392 ml]) can full-fat coconut milk, refrigerated for 24 hours

1 tablespoon (15 ml) maple syrup

1 pound (454 g) strawberries, hulled

¾ pound (340 g) blueberries

¾ pound (340 g) raspberries

1. Open the can of coconut milk without shaking it, and scoop out the cream sitting at the top of the can (the cream separates from the water when chilled). Add the cream to a bowl and stir in the maple syrup. Check for sweetness and adjust to taste.

To assemble: Divide the berries evenly among 5 containers. Top each serving with a dollop of coconut cream.

Note: Store for up to 5 days in an airtight container in the refrigerator. Not suitable for freezing.

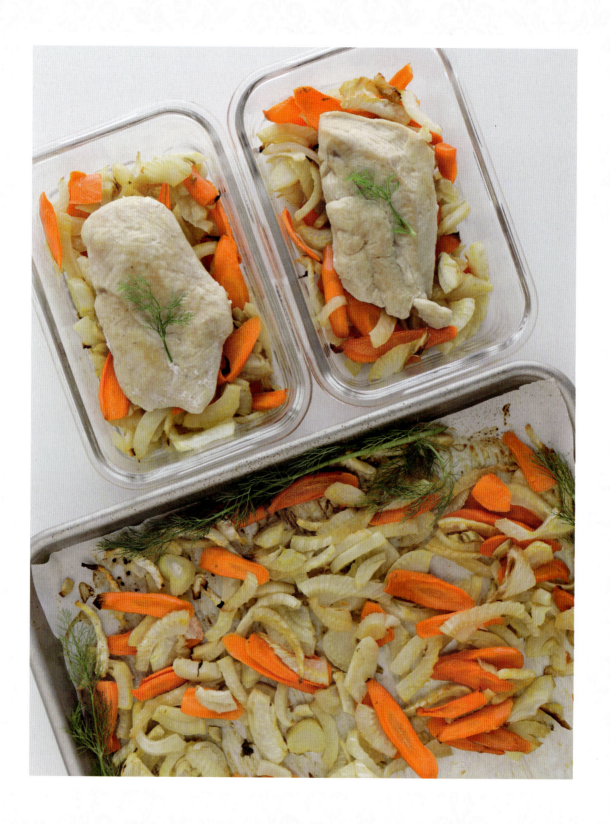

Chapter 8
LOW-CARB MEAL PLAN

You're sure to love this low-starch menu, even if you don't eat low carb all year-round. It's ideal as a post-holiday or post-celebration detox, as well as for general weight loss. And, as usual, it delivers on nutrients—via cauliflower, asparagus, mushrooms, and plenty of leafy greens instead of high-starch vegetables like sweet potatoes, parsnips, and winter squash.

You'll start your batch-cooking session with **Chicken with Roasted Fennel and Carrots**. Pair this beginner-friendly AIP meal with Quick Gravy for a little extra indulgence!

Because this week's focus is low carb, your snack is savory rather than sweet. **Savory Cauliflower Bites** will keep you going between meals: Make them with your favorite spice blends to change things up!

Then there's the **White Turkey Chili**. The bulk of this satiating white chili is made up of zucchini and kale, but I've added a small amount of white sweet potato to keep you from getting hungry too soon. Next comes another beginner-friendly AIP meal: **Pork Chops with Broccoli Mash** simple and wholesome, and so easy to pull together.

I've saved the best for last. This final recipe will blow your socks off for sure. My **Teriyaki Veggie Stir-Fry with Turmeric-Ginger Meatballs** is so much fun to eat and offers all the good feels of a great takeout meal—but it's full of antioxidants, nutrient-rich vegetables, and healthy protein, which means it's absolutely guilt-free!

Kitchen note: Make sure you have 1 quart (1 L) of chicken Bone Broth ready for your batch-cooking session.

	BREAKFAST	LUNCH	DINNER	SNACK
DAY 1	White Turkey Chili	Chicken with Roasted Fennel and Carrots	Teriyaki Veggie Stir-Fry with Turmeric-Ginger Meatballs	Savory Cauliflower Bites
DAY 2	Pork Chops with Broccoli Mash	White Turkey Chili	Chicken with Roasted Fennel and Carrots	Savory Cauliflower Bites
DAY 3	Teriyaki Veggie Stir-Fry with Turmeric-Ginger Meatballs	Pork Chops with Broccoli Mash	White Turkey Chili	Savory Cauliflower Bites
DAY 4	Chicken with Roasted Fennel and Carrots	Teriyaki Veggie Stir-Fry with Turmeric-Ginger Meatballs	Pork Chops with Broccoli Mash	Savory Cauliflower Bites
DAY 5	White Turkey Chili	Chicken with Roasted Fennel and Carrots	Teriyaki Veggie Stir-Fry with Turmeric-Ginger Meatballs	Savory Cauliflower Bites

EXTRA SERVINGS: 1 White Turkey Chili +
1 Teriyaki Veggie Stir-Fry with Turmeric-Ginger Meatballs + 1 Pork Chops with Broccoli Mash

Shopping List

PRODUCE

4 cloves garlic

¼ cup (60 ml) freshly squeezed lemon juice

½ red onion (⅓ pound [150 g])

1 bunch lacinato kale (½ pound [227 g])

1 yellow onion (¾ pound [340 g])

1 pound (454 g) broccoli florets

1 pound (454 g) mushrooms

4 carrots (10 ounces [280 g]) + ¾ pound (340 g) carrots

2 white sweet potatoes (1 pound + ¾ pound [454 g + 340 g])

4 zucchini (1¾ pounds [795 g])

2 bunches young green asparagus (2 pounds [908 g])

3 fennel bulbs (2 pounds [908 g])

1 head cauliflower (2½ pounds [1135 g])

MEAT/SEAFOOD

1 quart (1 L) chicken Bone Broth (page 180)

1 pound (454 g) ground turkey

1½ pounds (680 g) chicken breast cutlets (or see page 97 for how to make cutlets from chicken breasts)

1½ pounds (680 g) ground pork

4 thick boneless pork loin chops (1½ pounds [680 g])

HERBS AND SPICES

½ teaspoon ground turmeric

1 teaspoon onion powder

1 teaspoon dried thyme

1½ teaspoons garlic powder

1½ teaspoons ginger powder

¾ tablespoon dried basil

1 tablespoon (2 g) dried oregano

PANTRY ITEMS

1 tablespoon (8 g) arrowroot flour

2 tablespoons (16 g) coconut flour

¼ cup (60 ml) maple syrup

½ cup (120 ml) full-fat coconut milk

1 cup (235 ml) coconut aminos

OTHER

Coconut oil

Extra-virgin olive oil

Sea salt

Equipment and Tools

15 containers for your meals + 5 containers for
     snacks (see pages 32 to 33)

2 large rimmed baking sheets (12 x 17 inches
     [30.5 x 43 cm])

chef's knife

cutting board

food processor with S-blade

large skillet (at least 11 inches [28 cm] wide)

measuring cups and spoons

mixing bowl

parchment paper

pots and pans

resealable 1-gallon (3.6 L) plastic bags

stockpot

vegetable peeler

whisk

wooden spoon

Batch-Cooking Directions

1. Reminder: *The morning before*, defrost the meat if frozen. Make sure you have 1 quart (1 L) of chicken **Bone Broth** (page 180) on hand. Prepare your containers.

2. Preheat the oven to 400°F (200°C or gas mark 6). Place one rack in the middle and one rack at the bottom (second to the last slot) of the oven. Line two rimmed baking sheets with parchment paper.

3. Start your batch-cooking session with the **Chicken with Roasted Fennel and Carrots** (page 97), steps 1 through 4, placing the vegetables in the middle of the oven. Set a timer for 60 minutes.

4. Complete the **Savory Cauliflower Bites** (page 99), steps 1 through 5, placing the cauliflower at the bottom of the oven. Set a timer for 30 minutes. When the timer goes off, assemble.

5. When the timer goes off for the fennel and carrots, remove from the oven, set aside, complete step 5 of the **Chicken with Roasted Fennel and Carrots** (page 97), and assemble.

6. Complete the **White Turkey Chili** (page 100), steps 1 through 5, and assemble.

7. Complete the **Pork Chops with Broccoli Mash** (page 103), steps 1 and 2, and assemble.

8. Complete the **Teriyaki Veggie Stir-Fry with Turmeric-Ginger Meatballs** (page 104), steps 1 through 7, and assemble.

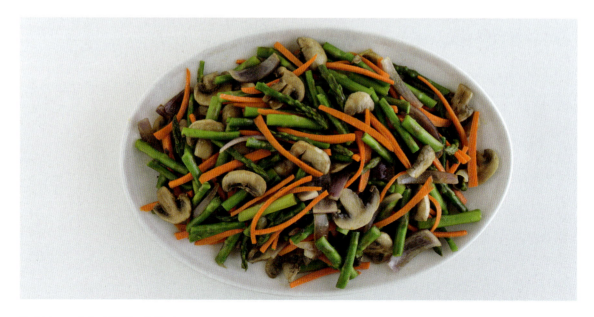

CHICKEN *with* ROASTED FENNEL *and* CARROTS

Fennel bulb has been valued since ancient times for its anti-inflammatory, antiviral, and antimicrobial properties—and it's especially delicious when roasted. It has a slight licorice or aniseed taste and pairs well with carrots and chicken in this no-fuss, low-carb recipe. Go ahead and enjoy fennel bulb, but remember that fennel seeds are not AIP compliant and should be avoided during the elimination phase.

Prep time:
15 minutes
Cook time:
1 hour
Yield:
4 servings

1½ pounds (680 g) chicken breast

3 fennel bulbs (2 pounds [908 g])

¾ pound (340 g) carrots

¼ cup (60 ml) freshly squeezed lemon juice

3 tablespoons (45 ml) coconut oil, divided

2 tablespoons (30 ml) maple syrup

1½ teaspoons sea salt, divided

1. Preheat the oven to 400°F (200°C or gas mark 6) and place the rack in the middle. Line a large rimmed baking sheet with parchment paper.

2. To cut chicken breasts into cutlets, use a chef's knife or paring knife to slice the breast horizontally into two even pieces. Pound them flat, then slice into 1-inch (2.5 cm) strips.

3. Cut off and discard the tops and bottoms of the fennel bulbs, then core and thinly slice. Peel and slice the carrots. Spread the prepared vegetables in a single layer on the baking sheet.

4. Add the lemon juice to a small bowl, plus 2 tablespoons (30 ml) of the coconut oil, melted, and the maple syrup. Stir and pour over the vegetables. Season with 1 teaspoon of the salt. Roast in the oven until tender, about 1 hour, tossing the vegetables a few times during roasting.

5. Meanwhile, pat the cutlets dry with a paper towel and season with the remaining ½ teaspoon salt on both sides. Heat the remaining 1 tablespoon (15 ml) coconut oil in a large skillet over medium heat. When hot, add the chicken and cook, covered, until no longer pink and the juices run clear, about 5 minutes on each side.

To assemble: Divide the ingredients evenly among 4 containers, starting with a layer of vegetables at the bottom and topping each with a piece of chicken.

Note: Store for up to 5 days in an airtight container in the refrigerator, or freeze for up to 4 months.

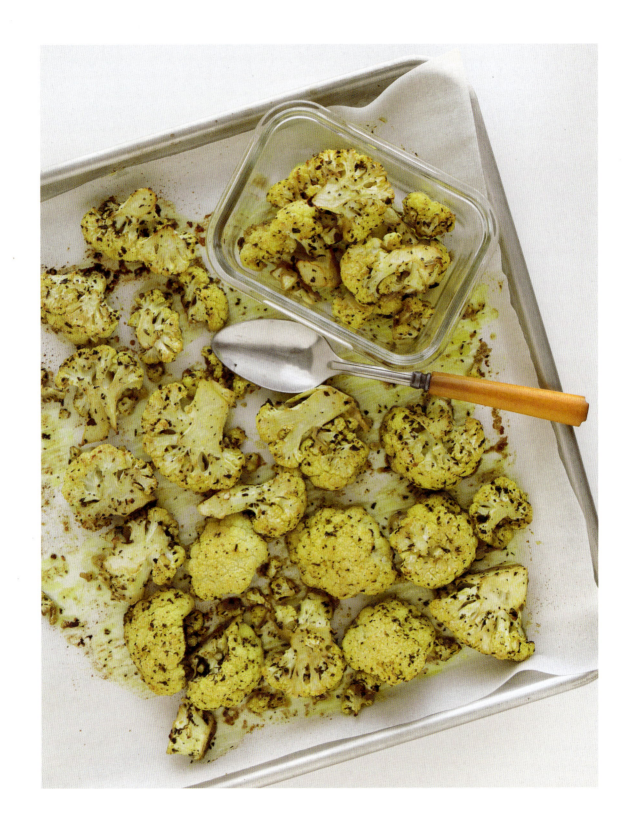

SAVORY CAULIFLOWER BITES

These addictive cauliflower bites, perfectly seasoned and slow-roasted in the oven, make a satisfying, guilt-free, low-carb snack that's also AIP friendly (they're like a healthier version of popcorn!). I use a blend of Middle Eastern–inspired spices in this recipe, but feel free to experiment with any of your favorite AIP-compliant herbs and spices (see page 17 for a complete list).

Prep time:
10 minutes
Cook time:
30 minutes
Yield:
5 servings

1 head cauliflower (2½ pounds [1135 g])

⅓ cup (80 ml) olive oil

2 tablespoons (30 ml) coconut aminos

¾ tablespoon dried basil

½ teaspoon garlic powder

½ teaspoon onion powder

¼ teaspoon ground turmeric

¼ teaspoon sea salt

1. Preheat the oven to 400°F (200°C or gas mark 6) and place the rack in the middle (or at the bottom if you are following the batch-cooking directions). Line a large rimmed baking sheet with parchment paper.

2. Discard all the green leaves from the cauliflower, cut off the excess stem, then cut the head into ¾-inch (2 cm) slices. Separate the slices into smaller pieces and transfer to a large resealable plastic bag.

3. Combine the olive oil, coconut aminos, basil, garlic powder, onion powder, turmeric, and salt in a small bowl. Mix well.

4. Sprinkle the spice mixture over the cauliflower. Seal the bag and massage until all the pieces are well coated.

5. Spread the cauliflower on the baking sheet in a single layer. Bake in the oven until golden brown and tender, 25 to 30 minutes.

   To assemble: Divide the cauliflower evenly among 5 containers.

   Note: Store for up to 5 days in an airtight container in the refrigerator, or freeze for up to 4 months.

WHITE TURKEY CHILI

This low-carb chili skips the traditional cannellini beans and dairy found in mainstream chili recipes. Loaded with health-promoting vegetables like zucchini, onions, kale, and white sweet potatoes plus easy-to-digest ground turkey, this white chili delivers a light and well-balanced meal—and it doesn't skimp on flavor, thanks to the fresh garlic and oregano. Who needs chile peppers, anyway?

Prep time:
15 minutes
Cook time:
20 minutes
Yield:
5 [16-ounce [454 g]] servings

4 zucchini (1¾ pounds [795 g])

1 yellow onion (¾ pound [340 g])

1 white sweet potato (1 pound [454 g])

1 bunch lacinato kale (½ pound [227 g])

4 cloves garlic

5 tablespoons (75 ml) olive oil, divided

1 pound (454 g) ground turkey

1¾ teaspoons sea salt, divided

1 quart (1 L) chicken Bone Broth (page 180)

1 tablespoon (2 g) dried oregano

1. Cut off and discard the tops and bottoms of the zucchini, then dice. Dice the onion. Peel and dice the sweet potato. Cut off and discard the hard stem at the bottom of the kale, then thinly slice the rest. Mince the garlic cloves.

2. Heat 2 tablespoons (30 ml) of the olive oil in a stockpot over medium heat. When hot, add the ground turkey and ¾ teaspoon of the salt, and cook until no longer pink, about 5 minutes. Transfer to a plate and return the pot to the heat.

3. Heat the remaining 3 tablespoons (45 ml) olive oil. When hot, add the onion, sweet potato, and garlic. Cover and cook for 10 minutes, stirring occasionally and making sure the vegetables don't stick to the bottom of the pot. If this happens, add ¼ cup (60 ml) of chicken broth.

4. Add the chicken broth, zucchini, and oregano. Cover and bring to a boil over high heat, then reduce the heat to medium and continue to cook until the vegetables are tender, about 5 minutes.

5. Remove the pot from the heat. Add the cooked turkey, kale, and remaining 1 teaspoon salt. Mix well, cover with the lid, and let rest for 5 minutes. Check the seasoning and adjust the salt to taste.

To assemble: Divide the White Turkey Chili evenly among 5 glass containers (or jars).

Note: Store for up to 5 days in an airtight container in the refrigerator, or freeze for up to 4 months.

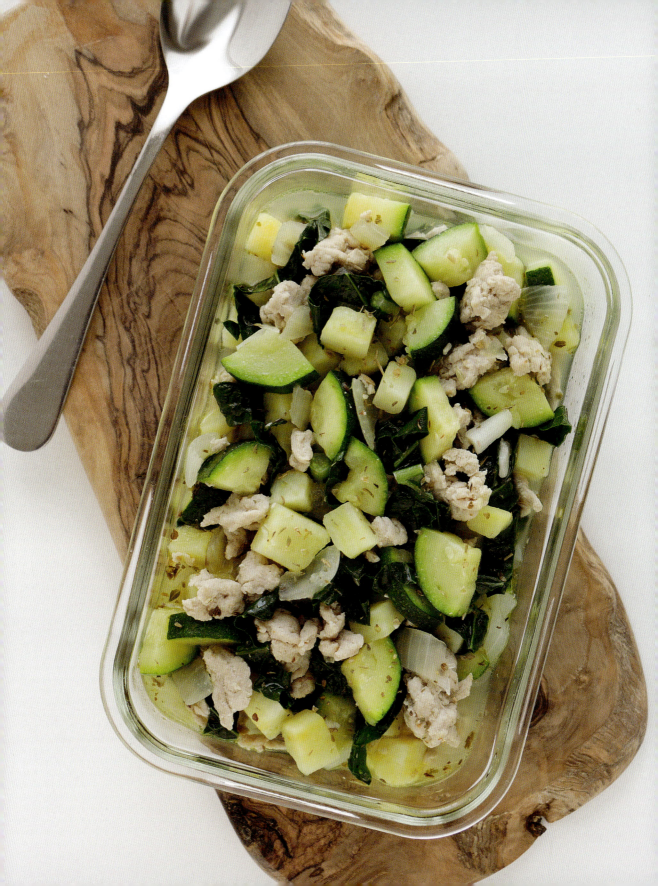

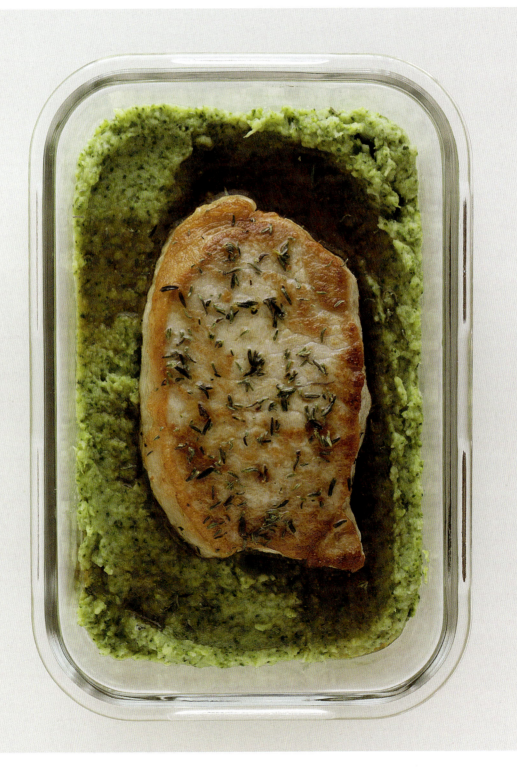

PORK CHOPS *with* BROCCOLI MASH

This meal scores a perfect ten on the comfort food scale, and it's so easy to prepare! Besides, it's incredibly nutritious. The creamy broccoli mash delivers a hefty dose of vitamins C and K, plus B vitamins and manganese, while the perfectly seared pork chops provide satiating protein.

Prep time:
7 minutes

Cook time:
15 minutes

Yield:
4 servings

1 recipe Broccoli Mash (page 181)

2 tablespoons (30 ml) olive oil

4 thick boneless pork loin chops
(1½ pounds [680 g])

1 teaspoon dried thyme

½ teaspoon sea salt

1. Prepare the Broccoli Mash following the directions on page 181.

2. While the vegetables are cooking, heat the olive oil over medium-high heat in a large skillet. Season the pork chops on both sides with the thyme and salt. When the oil is hot, sear the chops on both sides until golden brown, about 2 minutes on each side. Remove from the heat, cover with a lid, and let rest until you are finished making the Broccoli Mash.

To assemble: Divide the ingredients evenly among 4 glass containers. Start with a layer of broccoli mash at the bottom, then top with a pork chop. Drizzle the meat with leftover cooking juices.

Note: Store for up to 5 days in an airtight container in the refrigerator, or freeze for up to 4 months.

TERIYAKI VEGGIE STIR-FRY *with* TURMERIC-GINGER MEATBALLS

I'm absolutely in love with this meal, and I can't decide whether it was the brightly colored vegetables or the oh-so-tasty turmeric-ginger meatballs with their flavorful teriyaki sauce that won me over in the first place! A note about the vegetables: If you can't source young, thin asparagus for this recipe and end up with "adult" asparagus (thicker than ⅓ inch [8 mm] in diameter), extend its cooking time by about 5 minutes until the spears are crisp-tender.

Prep time:
30 minutes
Cook time:
30 minutes
Yield:
5 servings

2 bunches young green asparagus (2 pounds [908 g])

1 pound (454 g) mushrooms

4 carrots (10 ounces [280 g])

½ red onion (about ⅓ pound [150 g])

5 tablespoons (75 ml) olive oil, divided

1½ pounds (680 g) ground pork

2 tablespoons (30 ml) coconut aminos

2 tablespoons (16 g) coconut flour

¾ teaspoon sea salt, plus more to taste

½ teaspoon ginger powder

¼ teaspoon ground turmeric

1 recipe Teriyaki Sauce (page 186)

1. Cut off and discard the woody ends of the asparagus (about 1½ inches [3.8 cm]), then slice into 1½-inch (3.8 cm) long pieces. Slice the mushrooms. Peel and julienne the carrots. Chop the onion.

2. Heat 2 tablespoons (30 ml) of the olive oil in a large skillet over medium heat. When hot, add the mushrooms. Cover and cook until crisp-tender, about 5 minutes. Transfer to a large bowl and return the skillet to the heat.

3. Heat 1 tablespoon (15 ml) of the olive oil in the skillet and add the asparagus. Cover and cook until crisp-tender, about 5 minutes. Transfer to the large bowl with the mushrooms and return the skillet to the heat.

4. Heat 1 tablespoon (15 ml) of olive oil in the skillet, then add the carrots and onion. Cover and cook until crisp-tender, about 4 minutes. Transfer to the large bowl and wipe the skillet clean.

5. In a separate bowl, combine the ground pork, coconut aminos, coconut flour, salt, ginger, and turmeric. Mix thoroughly using your hands, then form into 1-inch (2.5 cm) meatballs to obtain 30 meatballs.

6. Heat the remaining 1 tablespoon (15 ml) olive oil in the skillet over medium heat. When hot, add the meatballs and cook, covered, until no longer pink inside, about 12 minutes, flipping them halfway through.

7. While the meatballs are cooking, prepare the Teriyaki Sauce (page 186). Pour the sauce over the vegetables (reserving ¼ cup [60 ml]), mix well using two large spoons, and add salt to taste.

To assemble: Divide the ingredients evenly among 5 glass containers, starting with a layer of vegetables at the bottom, and topping each with 6 meatballs. Finish each with a drizzle of the reserved Teriyaki Sauce.

Note: Store for up to 5 days in an airtight container in the refrigerator, or freeze for up to 4 months.

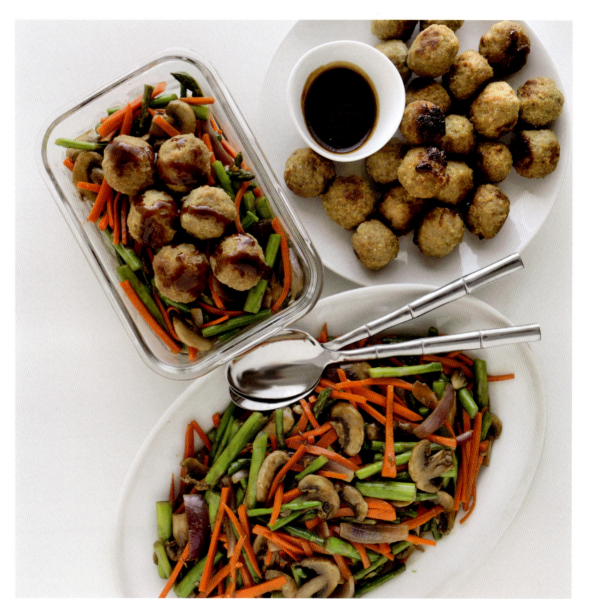

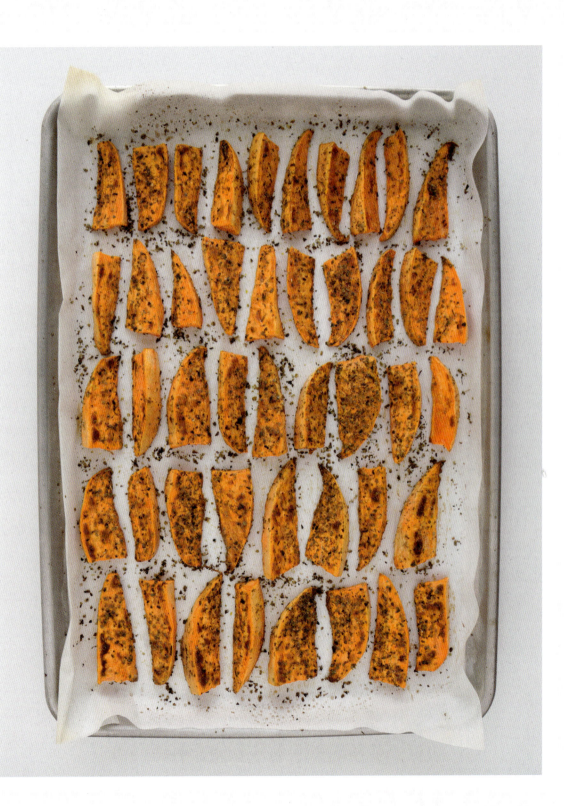

Chapter 9

COCONUT-FREE MEAL PLAN

All coconut products are AIP compliant and incredibly versatile. Coconut milk, with its rich and creamy texture, is a wonderful dairy-free replacement for cow's milk, while coconut aminos can stand in for soy sauce in recipes like stir-fries and Asian dishes. Coconut products are also widely used in AIP-friendly desserts and baked goods. But, while coconut is a nutrient-dense superfood, it can be a gut irritant for some people. In that case, it's best avoided.

This chapter will show you how easy that can be. Coconut might be missing from this week's meal plan, but yummy and nutritious are very much on the menu! The **Skirt Steak with Seasoned Sweet Potato Wedges and Broccoli** is a classic I can't get enough of. (Who can say no to baked fries, right?!) Just try not to eat them all before they even make it to the table!

Next, get ready for a phenomenal **Teriyaki Pineapple Chicken**. This one-pan wonder boasts a seriously addictive (and, of course, AIP-compliant) Teriyaki Sauce. Use it to complement your stir-fries or to whip up party-ready Teriyaki Chicken Wings.

Southwestern-inspired **Steak Salad with Jicama-Mango Salsa** is excellent as a quick lunch option at home, at work, or anywhere on the go. And my **Turkey Patties with Cauliflower Rice and Collard Greens** is my version of AIP soul food: It's a simple, nutritious, and well-balanced meal that will keep you nourished for hours at a time.

Have you ever made **Tostones**? If not, you'll thank me for this week's snack! This snack is a great all-rounder: Whether you choose to pair it with something sweet (a piece of fruit) or savory (mashed avocado), it's always satisfyingly crunchy (and fun and easy to make).

	BREAKFAST	LUNCH	DINNER	SNACK
DAY 1	Turkey Patties with Cauliflower Rice and Collard Greens	Steak Salad with Jicama-Mango Salsa	Skirt Steak with Seasoned Sweet Potato Wedges and Broccoli	Tostones
DAY 2	Teriyaki Pineapple Chicken	Steak Salad with Jicama-Mango Salsa	Turkey Patties with Cauliflower Rice and Collard Greens	Tostones
DAY 3	Turkey Patties with Cauliflower Rice and Collard Greens	Skirt Steak with Seasoned Sweet Potato Wedges and Broccoli	Steak Salad with Jicama-Mango Salsa	Tostones
DAY 4	Skirt Steak with Seasoned Sweet Potato Wedges and Broccoli	Steak Salad with Jicama-Mango Salsa	Teriyaki Pineapple Chicken	Tostones
DAY 5	Skirt Steak with Seasoned Sweet Potato Wedges and Broccoli	Turkey Patties with Cauliflower Rice and Collard Greens	Teriyaki Pineapple Chicken	Tostones

EXTRA SERVINGS: 1 Teriyaki Pineapple Chicken +
1 Turkey Patties with Cauliflower Rice and Collard Greens

Shopping List

PRODUCE

1 lime

2 tablespoons (30 ml) freshly squeezed
    lemon juice

¼ cup (5 g) packed minced cilantro

⅓ cup (80 ml) orange juice

1 yellow onion (10 ounces [280 g])

1 jicama (¾ pound [340 g])

1 mango (¾ pound [340 g])

1 red onion (¾ pound [340 g])

¾ pound (340 g) broccoli florets

1 pound (454 g) mushrooms

1 pound (454 g) romaine lettuce

2 (8-ounce [227 g]) bunches collard greens

1 head cauliflower (2 pounds [908 g])

2 sweet potatoes (1½ pounds [680 g])

3 green plantains

4 baby bok choy (1½ pounds [680 g])

MEAT/SEAFOOD

1¼ pounds (568 g) boneless skinless chicken
    breasts

1¼ pounds (568 g) ground turkey

2 pounds (908 g) skirt flank steak
    (or similar cut)

HERBS AND SPICES

¼ teaspoon dried cilantro

1 teaspoon ginger powder

1 teaspoon dried marjoram

1¼ teaspoons garlic powder

1¾ teaspoons onion powder

PANTRY ITEMS

1 teaspoon honey

1 tablespoon (8 g) arrowroot flour

2 tablespoons (30 ml) maple syrup

¾ cup (180 ml) coconut aminos

1 cup (235 ml) avocado oil

1 (20-ounce [560 g]) can pineapple chunks

OTHER

Coconut oil

Extra-virgin olive oil

Sea salt

Equipment and Tools

15 containers for your meals + 5 containers for snacks (see pages 32 to 33)

2 large rimmed baking sheets (12 x 17 inches [30.5 x 43 cm])

chef's knife

cutting board

food processor with S-blade

large skillet (at least 11 inches [28 cm] wide)

measuring cups and spoons

mixing bowls of different sizes

saucepan

slotted spatula

vegetable peeler

whisk

wooden spoon

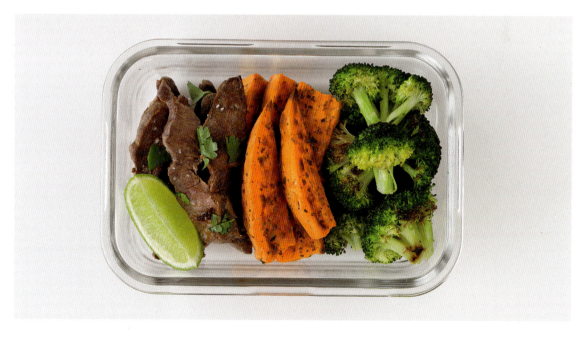

Batch-Cooking Directions

1. Reminder: *The morning before*, defrost the meat if frozen. Prepare your containers.

2. Start your batch-cooking session with the **Skirt Steak with Seasoned Sweet Potato Wedges and Broccoli** (page 111), steps 1 through 3. Set one timer for 20 minutes and another timer for 50 minutes. While both vegetables are cooking, cut all the skirt flank steak into ½-inch (1 cm) strips, but don't start cooking the meat yet. Measure out 1¼ pounds (568 g) of steak and separate it from the remaining ¾ pound (340 g) because you will use the meat in two different recipes.

3. When the timer goes off for the broccoli, transfer it to a plate and line the baking sheet with fresh parchment paper. Also, flip the sweet potato wedges over.

4. Start cooking the skirt steak following the directions on page 111, step 4, keeping the meat for the two recipes separate.

5. When the timer goes off for the sweet potato wedges, transfer them to a plate and line the baking sheet with fresh parchment paper.

6. Complete the **Teriyaki Pineapple Chicken** (page 113), steps 1 through 5. Set one timer for 30 minutes and another timer for 40 minutes. Meanwhile, complete the **Steak Salad with Jicama-Mango Salsa** (page 114), steps 2 through 4.

7. Now take a breather and assemble the **Skirt Steak with Seasoned Sweet Potato Wedges and Broccoli** (page 111), the **Teriyaki Pineapple Chicken** (page 113), and the **Steak Salad with Jicama-Mango Salsa** (page 114).

8. Complete the **Turkey Patties with Cauliflower Rice and Collard Greens** (page 117), steps 1 through 4, and assemble.

9. Finish your batch-cooking session with the **Tostones** (page 118), steps 1 through 4, and assemble.

SKIRT STEAK *with* SEASONED SWEET POTATO WEDGES *and* BROCCOLI

I never get tired of steak and fries: It's one of my favorite treats! But I've learned how to make it much healthier, swapping deep-fried, potato-based fries for oven-baked sweet potato wedges. I think they're even better than the regular version, especially when seasoned with AIP-approved spices! A side of nutrient-rich roasted broccoli rounds this meal off perfectly.

Prep time:
10 minutes
Cook time:
50 minutes
Yield:
4 servings

2 sweet potatoes (about 1½ pounds [680 g])

¾ pound (340 g) broccoli florets

3 tablespoons (30 ml) avocado oil, divided

1½ teaspoons sea salt, divided

1 teaspoon dried marjoram

1 teaspoon onion powder

1¼ pounds (680 g) skirt flank steak

1. Preheat the oven to 400°F (200°C or gas mark 6). Place one rack in the middle and one rack at the bottom of the oven. Line two baking sheets with parchment paper.

2. Peel and cut the sweet potato into wedges. In a mixing bowl, combine the sweet potato wedges, broccoli florets, 2 tablespoons (30 ml) of the avocado oil, and 1 teaspoon of the salt. Mix well using your hands. Arrange the seasoned sweet potato wedges on a baking sheet in a single layer (don't let them overlap). Sprinkle with the marjoram and onion powder. Arrange the broccoli florets on the other baking sheet.

3. Place the broccoli at the bottom of the oven and roast for 20 minutes. Place the sweet potatoes in the middle of the oven and roast for 50 minutes, turning them over halfway, until cooked through and nicely browned.

4. Meanwhile, slice the skirt steak into ½-inch (1 cm) strips. Heat the remaining 1 tablespoon (15 ml) avocado oil in a large nonstick skillet over medium-high heat. Add the steak and the remaining ½ teaspoon salt. Sear for 2 to 3 minutes, stirring a few times, until the strips are cooked on all sides (you may want to use a lid to avoid splattering). They will still be slightly pink inside. Transfer the meat to a plate with a slotted spatula.

To assemble: Divide the sweet potato wedges, broccoli, and steak evenly among 4 containers.

Note: Store for up to 5 days in an airtight container in the refrigerator, or freeze for up to 4 months.

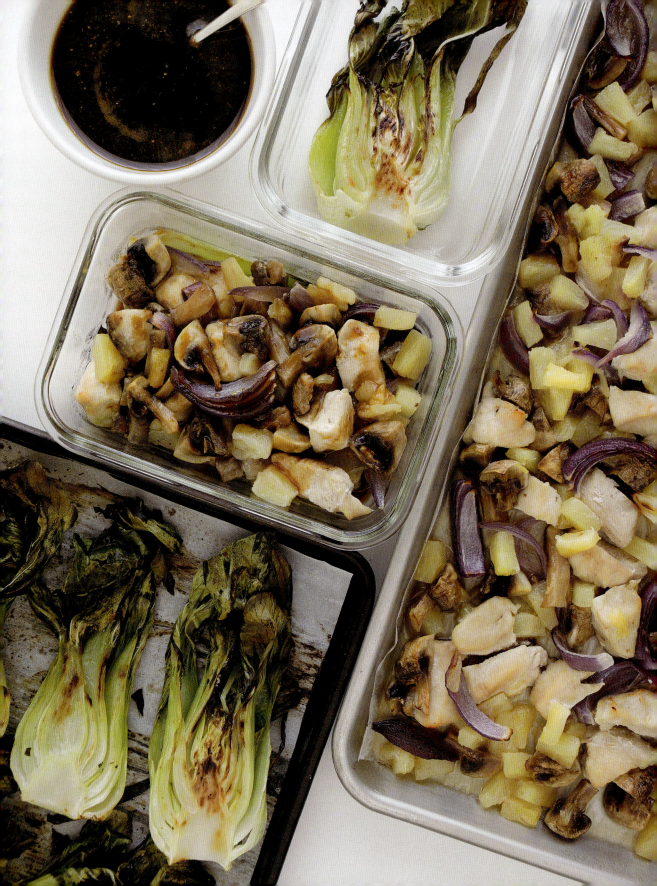

TERIYAKI PINEAPPLE CHICKEN

This quick, Asian-inspired meal is basically an oven-roasted stir-fry. All you need to do is grab a handful of ingredients plus a couple AIP-friendly staples: Then you can let your oven do the rest of the work for you! Pro tip: When choosing the pineapple, be sure to look for canned pineapple chunks with no added sugar or citric acid.

Prep time:
20 minutes

Cook time:
40 minutes

Yield:
4 servings

4 baby bok choy (1½ pounds [680 g])

¼ cup (60 ml) avocado oil, divided

2½ teaspoons sea salt, divided

1¼ pounds (568 g) boneless skinless chicken breasts

1 pound (454 g) mushrooms

1 red onion (½ pound [227 g])

1 (20-ounce [560 g]) can pineapple chunks, drained

1 recipe Teriyaki Sauce (page 186)

1. Preheat the oven to 400°F (200°C or gas mark 6). Place one rack in the middle and one rack on the second-to-last slot from the bottom of the oven. Line two rimmed baking sheets with parchment paper.

2. Cut the baby bok choy in half lengthwise and spread them on one of the baking sheets, cut-side up. Drizzle with 2 tablespoons (30 ml) of the avocado oil and season with ½ teaspoon of the salt.

3. Dice the chicken breasts into 1-inch (2.5 cm) pieces. Quarter the mushrooms and chop the onion. Combine the chicken, mushrooms, onion, and pineapple chunks in a large bowl. Drizzle with the remaining 2 tablespoons (30 ml) avocado oil and season with the remaining 2 teaspoons salt. Mix well. Spread on the other baking sheet.

4. Place the bok choy at the bottom of the oven and cook for 30 minutes, flipping them over halfway through. Place the chicken mixture in the middle of the oven and cook for 40 minutes.

5. Meanwhile, prepare the Teriyaki Sauce following the recipe on page 186.

To assemble: Divide the ingredients evenly among 4 containers, starting with 2 pieces of bok choy at the bottom and topping each with a quarter of the chicken mixture. Finish each with a serving of Teriyaki Sauce.

Note: Store for up to 5 days in an airtight container in the refrigerator, or freeze for up to 4 months.

STEAK SALAD WITH JICAMA-MANGO SALSA

Lively, cilantro-rich jicama-mango salsa takes center stage in this southwestern-inspired salad and acts as a sweet and tangy counterpart to tender pieces of skirt steak. Topped with a citrusy vinaigrette, this salad makes an ideal light lunch or dinner—and it's sure to impress your guests, too!

Prep time:
25 minutes
Cook time:
6 minutes
Yield:
4 servings

¾ pound (340 g) skirt steak

1 tablespoon (15 ml) avocado oil

¼ teaspoon sea salt

1 pound (454 g) romaine lettuce

1 jicama (¾ pound [340 g])

1 mango (¾ pound [340 g])

½ red onion (4 ounces [112 g])

¼ cup (5 g) packed minced cilantro

Juice of 1 lime

Vinaigrette (page 185)

1. Slice the skirt steak into ½-inch (1 cm) strips. Heat the avocado oil in a large nonstick skillet over medium-high heat. Add the steak and season with the salt. Sear for 2 to 3 minutes, stirring occasionally, until the steak strips are cooked on all sides. They will still be slightly pink inside. Transfer the meat to a plate with a slotted spatula and let cool.

2. Thinly slice the romaine lettuce. Peel and dice the jicama into ¼-inch (6 mm) pieces. Do the same for the mango and red onion.

3. In a large bowl, combine the jicama, mango, red onion, cilantro, and lime juice. Mix well.

4. Prepare the Vinaigrette on page 185.

   To assemble: Divide the ingredients evenly among 4 containers or glass jars, starting with the jicama-mango salsa at the bottom, followed by the skirt steak and then the romaine lettuce. I prefer to keep the dressing on the side and add it at the last minute, right before serving. This helps keep the salad looking fresher for longer.

   Note: Store for up to 5 days in an airtight container in the refrigerator. Not suitable for freezing.

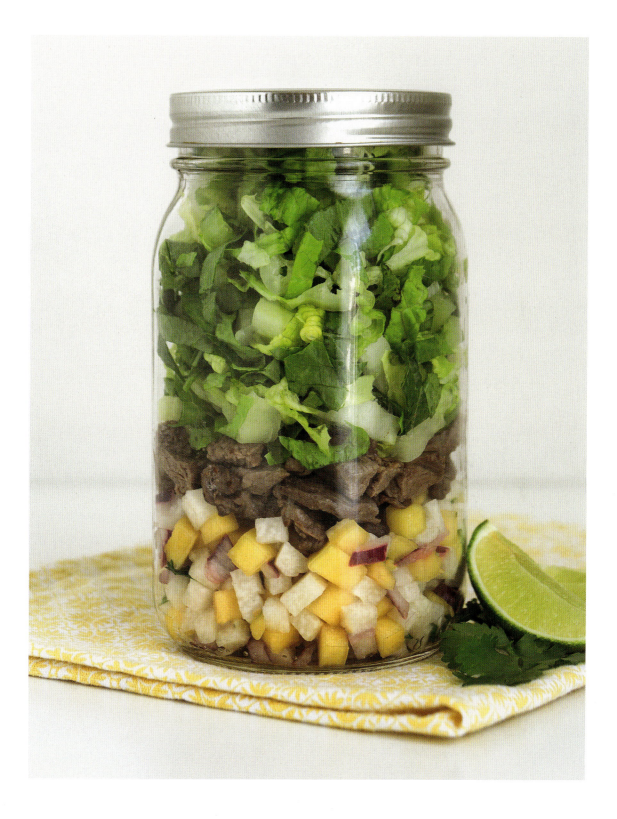

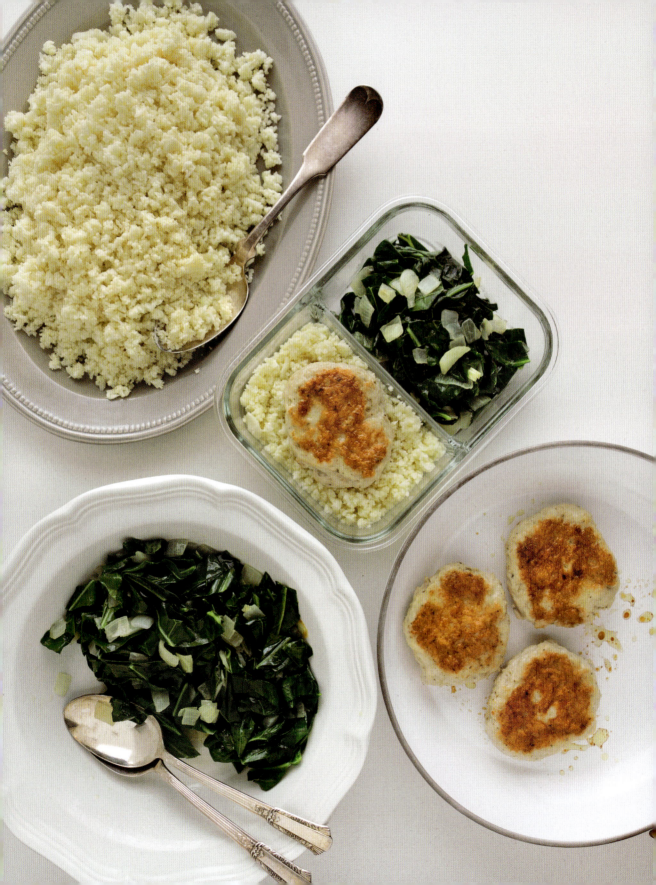

TURKEY PATTIES *with* CAULIFLOWER RICE *and* COLLARD GREENS

This is my kind of meal: uncomplicated and no fuss, with a boatload of vegetables to boot. The result is a highly nutritious meal packed with vitamins, minerals, and antioxidants. And it's also incredibly versatile: Swap the collard greens for kale or chard, and experiment with different kinds of meat for the patties. Use this recipe as a template and change up the ingredients to suit your taste—or whatever happens to be on sale at the grocery store!

Prep time:
20 minutes
Cook time:
26 minutes
Yield:
5 servings

1 recipe Cauliflower Rice (page 177)

2 bunches collard greens (½ pound [227 g] each)

1 yellow onion (10 ounces [280 g])

5 tablespoons (75 ml) olive oil, divided, plus more as needed

1½ teaspoons sea salt, divided

1¼ pounds (568 g) ground turkey

¼ teaspoon garlic powder

¼ teaspoon onion powder

¼ teaspoon dried cilantro (or similar dried herb, such as parsley, basil, or oregano)

1. Prepare the Cauliflower Rice (page 177). While the cauliflower is cooking, remove and discard the hard stems from the collard greens, then slice the leaves into ½-inch (1 cm)-thick strips. Dice the onion.

2. Transfer the Cauliflower Rice to a plate and wipe the skillet clean. Heat 3 tablespoons (45 ml) of the olive oil over medium heat. When hot, add the onion and cook, covered, until translucent, about 5 minutes. Add the collard greens and ¼ teaspoon of the salt, and continue to cook, covered, until wilted, about 3 minutes. Transfer to a plate and wipe the skillet clean again.

3. In a large bowl, combine the ground turkey, remaining 1¼ teaspoons salt, garlic powder, onion powder, and dried cilantro. Using lightly oiled hands, mix thoroughly, divide the meat into 5 portions, and form into patties.

4. Heat the remaining 2 tablespoons (30 ml) olive oil in the skillet over medium heat. When hot, add the turkey patties and cook until golden, about 4 minutes on each side. (You may have to add more oil while cooking if the patties start to stick to the bottom of the skillet.)

To assemble: Divide the Cauliflower Rice, collard greens, and turkey patties evenly among 5 containers (you will have an extra portion of Cauliflower Rice).

Note: Store for up to 5 days in an airtight container in the refrigerator, or freeze for up to 4 months.

TOSTONES

Tostones, or fried green plantains, don't have a lot of taste by themselves (unlike bananas, they aren't sweet), so it's up to you to season them with your favorite herbs and spices, like sea salt, garlic powder, or onion powder—or even cinnamon! For an extra nutritious (and filling) snack that's full of good fats, make instant guacamole by mashing half an avocado and seasoning it with salt and a little bit of lemon or lime juice, and then use tostones to scoop it up.

Prep time:
15 minutes
Cook time:
30 minutes
Yield:
5 or 6 servings

3 green plantains

⅓ cup (80 ml) avocado oil or tallow

1. Cut off the tops and bottoms of the plantains and peel with a vegetable peeler. Slice the peeled plantains into 1-inch (2.5 cm)-thick pieces.

2. Heat the avocado oil in a large skillet over medium heat. When hot, add the plantain pieces in a single layer (don't let them overlap). Fry until golden, 3 minutes per side. You may have to do this in several batches.

3. Use a slotted spatula to transfer the cooked plantain pieces to a paper towel–lined plate. Let cool slightly, then place the plantain between two sheets of parchment paper and flatten each piece with the flat back of a measuring cup until it is ¼ inch (6 mm) thick.

4. Return the flattened plantain pieces to the hot skillet (again, in a single layer) and fry until crisp, 1 to 2 minutes on each side. Transfer to a paper towel–lined plate and drain the excess oil.

To assemble: Once completely cool, divide the Tostones evenly among 5 or 6 containers.

Note: Store for up to 5 days in an airtight container in the refrigerator. Not suitable for freezing.

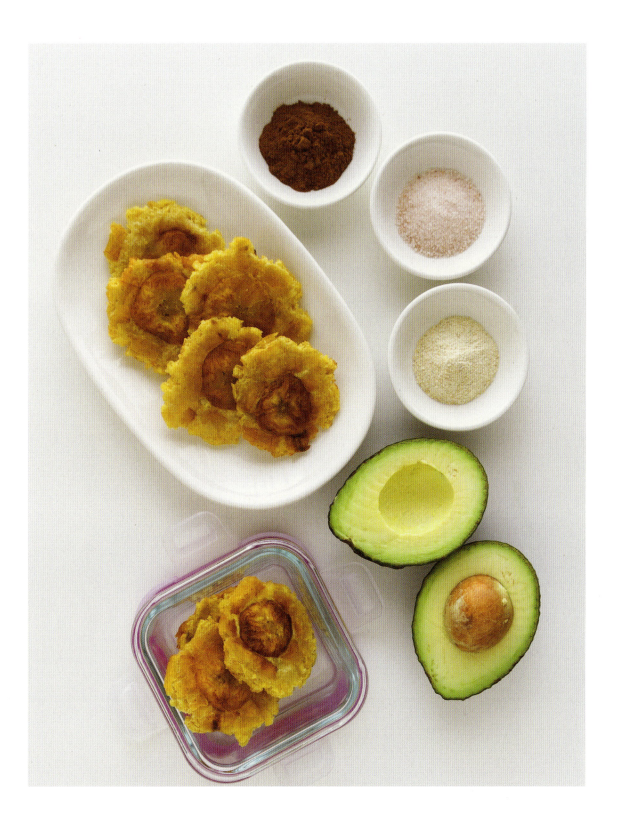

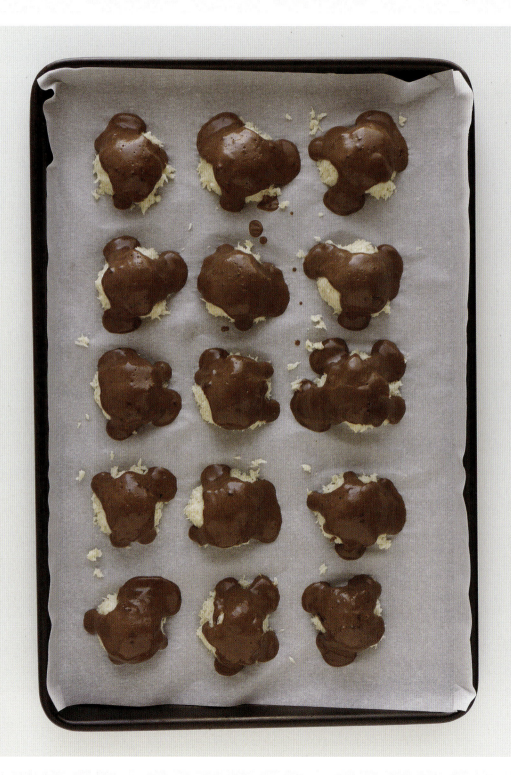

Chapter 10
FLAVORS OF THE WORLD MEAL PLAN

eady for a trip around the world? Your AIP menu this week will take you on an international culinary tour from France to Morocco to Vietnam and Thailand. We'll start your batch-cooking session with a nod to France with my guilt-free **No-Bake Macaroons with Chocolate Sauce**. The chocolate sauce might just be the best part: You can use it to top just about any other dessert, like ice cream or fresh fruit. (Just try not to eat the whole batch at once!)

Next on your menu is **Chicken Pho**. Served with zucchini noodles instead of rice noodles and full of tender chicken, this home-cooked Vietnamese soup gets a ton of flavor from its garnishes: fresh basil, sliced scallions, and delicate enoki mushrooms. Use chopsticks to help you slurp it up!

Then the **Moroccan Chicken with Butternut Squash Rice** brings you bright colors plus a bouquet of sweet and spicy aromas, all wrapped up in one neat little package. Don't skimp on the spices: Cinnamon, ginger, and cloves make this dish truly magical.

Quickly prepared and conveniently stored in a glass jar, the **Asian Steak Salad** makes the ideal portable lunch, whether you're at the office, in the car, on a picnic—or just about anywhere! Finally, my **Thai Curry Meatballs**, served with a side of Cauliflower Rice, will wow you with its rich, creamy, and mildly spicy curry sauce. (If you prefer your curry with lots of extra kick, play around with the amounts of fresh ginger, garlic, and/or lime juice.)

Kitchen note: Don't forget to prepare the marinade for the Asian Steak Salad the day before (see batch-cooking directions), and make sure you have 1½ quarts + ¾ cup (1.5 L + 180 ml) chicken Bone Broth on hand.

	BREAKFAST	LUNCH	DINNER	SNACK
DAY 1	Moroccan Chicken with Butternut Squash Rice	Asian Steak Salad	Thai Curry Meatballs	No-Bake Macaroons with Chocolate Sauce
DAY 2	Chicken Pho	Asian Steak Salad	Moroccan Chicken with Butternut Squash Rice	No-Bake Macaroons with Chocolate Sauce
DAY 3	Thai Curry Meatballs	Chicken Pho	Asian Steak Salad	No-Bake Macaroons with Chocolate Sauce
DAY 4	Chicken Pho	Asian Steak Salad	Thai Curry Meatballs	No-Bake Macaroons with Chocolate Sauce
DAY 5	Moroccan Chicken with Butternut Squash Rice	Thai Curry Meatballs	Chicken Pho	No-Bake Macaroons with Chocolate Sauce

EXTRA SERVINGS: 2 Moroccan Chicken with Butternut Squash Rice

Shopping List

PRODUCE

1 teaspoon grated fresh ginger

1 (3-inch [7.5 cm]) knob fresh ginger

1 bunch cilantro

1 head garlic

1 large pear

4 limes

4 scallions

1 ounce (28 g) fresh basil

2 tablespoons (8 g) minced fresh basil

⅓ cup (80 ml) freshly squeezed orange juice

1⅓ cups (150 g) shredded carrot

1 carrot (6 ounces [168 g])

6 ounces (168 g) shiitake mushrooms

½ pound (227 g) baby spinach

1 (10-ounce [280 g]) cucumber

1 butternut squash (2 pounds [908 g])

1 cauliflower head (2 pounds [908 g])

2 (1-pound [454 g]) sweet potatoes

2 (½-pound [227 g]) zucchini + 1 (6-ounce [168 g]) zucchini

3 (½-pound [227 g]) yellow onions

3½ ounces (100 g) enoki mushrooms

MEAT/SEAFOOD

¾ pound (340 g) skirt steak

1 pound (454 g) ground chicken

1½ quarts + ¾ cup (1.5 L + 180 ml) chicken Bone Broth (page 180)

2¼ pounds (1 kg) boneless skinless chicken breasts

HERBS AND SPICES

⅛ teaspoon ground cloves

½ teaspoon ground cinnamon

½ teaspoon ginger powder

PANTRY ITEMS

1 tablespoon (8 g) gelatin powder

2 tablespoons (16 g) roasted carob powder

2 tablespoons (30 ml) fish sauce

3 tablespoons (45 ml) maple syrup

4 tablespoons (60 ml) coconut aminos

4 tablespoons (80 g) honey

½ + ⅓ cup (120 + 80 ml) full-fat coconut milk

1 cup (110 g) pitted black olives

1 (14-ounce [392 ml]) can full-fat coconut milk

1 (15-ounce [420 g]) can sliced peaches

2 cups (170 g) unsweetened shredded coconut

OTHER

Coconut oil

Extra-virgin olive oil

Sea salt

Equipment and Tools

15 containers for your meals + 5 containers for snacks (see pages 32 to 33)

chef's knife

citrus press

cutting board

food processor with S-blade and shredding disk

ladle

large rimmed baking sheet (12 x 17 inches [30.5 x 43 cm])

large skillet (at least 11 inches [28 cm] wide)

measuring cups and spoons

mixing bowls

pots and pans

resealable plastic bag

slotted spatula

vegetable peeler

vegetable spiralizer

Batch-Cooking Directions

1. Reminder: *The morning before*, thaw the meat if frozen. *The day before*, prepare the marinade for the **Asian Steak Salad** (page 131, step 1). Make sure you have 1½ quarts + ¾ cup (1.5 L + 180 ml) chicken **Bone Broth** (page 180) on hand. Prepare your containers.

2. Start your batch-cooking session with the **No-Bake Macaroons with Chocolate Sauce** (page 125), steps 1 through 6, and refrigerate.

3. Complete the **Chicken Pho** (page 127), steps 1 through 4, and assemble.

4. Complete the **Moroccan Chicken with Butternut Squash Rice** (page 128), steps 1 through 4, and assemble.

5. Complete the **Asian Steak Salad** (page 131), steps 2 through 5, and assemble.

6. Finish your batch-cooking session with the **Thai Curry Meatballs** (page 132), steps 1 through 5, and assemble.

7. Don't forget to assemble the **No-Bake Macaroons with Chocolate Sauce** (page 125) in the refrigerator!

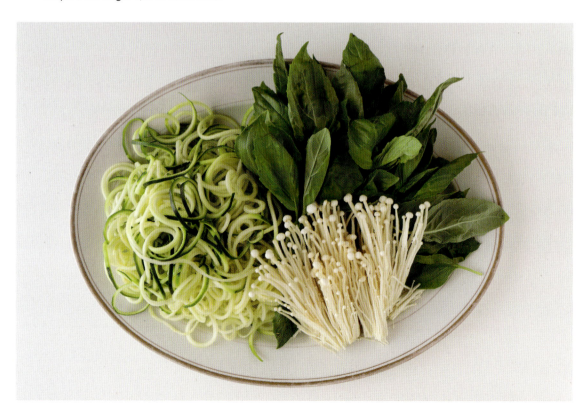

NO-BAKE MACAROONS *with* CHOCOLATE SAUCE

Skip the sugar and the egg whites in store-bought macaroons, and make them yourself with this simple no-bake recipe. You can mix the dough in a snap, then prepare the chocolate sauce while the macaroons cool in the refrigerator. And that's it: You're done! Next, get out your finest china, invite a friend over, and enjoy a chocolate-covered macaroon (or two, or three) over a cup of tea and some good conversation.

Prep time:
10 minutes
Cook time:
5 minutes
Yield:
15 macaroons

FOR THE MACAROONS:

⅓ cup (80 ml) full-fat coconut milk

3 tablespoons (60 g) honey

1 tablespoon (15 ml) coconut oil

3 tablespoons (45 ml) water
(at room temperature)

1 tablespoon (8 g) gelatin powder

2 cups (170 g) unsweetened shredded coconut

FOR THE CHOCOLATE SAUCE:

½ cup (120 ml) coconut milk

2 tablespoons (16 g) roasted carob
powder

1 tablespoon (15 ml) coconut oil

½ tablespoon honey

1. Line a baking sheet with parchment paper.

2. To make the macaroons, add the coconut milk, honey, and coconut oil to a small saucepan. Heat over medium heat while stirring until the ingredients are combined, about 2 minutes. Remove from the heat.

3. Combine the water and gelatin in a small cup. Stir well until the gelatin has dissolved and you obtain a gel-like mixture.

4. Pour the gelatin mixture into the saucepan and mix well. Stir in the shredded coconut until you obtain a crumbly coconut mixture.

5. Pack a measuring tablespoon tightly with the coconut mixture to form little tablespoon-size macaroons and transfer them to the baking sheet (use your finger or a regular spoon to help unmold the macaroon). You should have enough to make at least 15 macaroons. Refrigerate while you prepare the chocolate sauce.

6. To make the chocolate sauce, combine the coconut milk, carob powder, coconut oil, and honey in another small saucepan. Heat over medium heat while stirring until you obtain a smooth chocolate sauce, about 2 minutes. Drizzle over the macaroons and continue to refrigerate for 1 hour. Keep refrigerated until needed.

To assemble: Once the chocolate sauce is hardened, divide the macaroons evenly among 5 containers.

Note: Store for up to 5 days in an airtight container in the refrigerator. Not suitable for freezing.

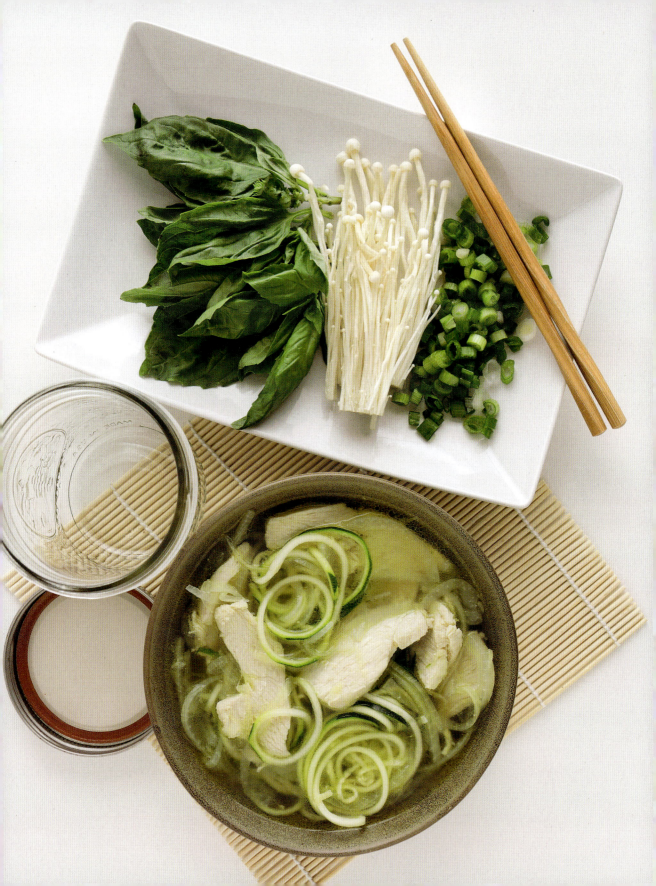

CHICKEN PHO

Inspired by traditional Vietnamese cuisine, this AIP-compliant pho gets its fabulous flavor from zucchini noodles, tender chicken, enoki mushrooms, scallions, and fresh basil. Don't worry if you have trouble sourcing enoki mushrooms; just replace them with sliced shiitake mushrooms, cooked following the directions in step 3 of the Asian Steak Salad (page 131).

Prep time:
12 minutes
Cook time:
10 minutes
Yield:
4 servings

1 (½-pound [227 g]) yellow onion

1-inch (2.5 cm) knob fresh ginger

1 pound (454 g) boneless skinless chicken breasts

2 (½-pound [227 g]) zucchini

4 scallions

2 tablespoons (30 ml) coconut oil

1½ quarts (1.5 L) chicken Bone Broth (page 180)

¾ teaspoon salt

3½ ounces (100 g) enoki mushrooms

1 ounce (28 g) fresh basil

1. Thinly slice the onion. Peel and grate the ginger. Slice the chicken into ¼-inch (6 mm) strips. Spiralize the zucchini to make noodles. Thinly slice the scallions.

2. Heat the coconut oil in a stockpot over medium heat. Add the onions and ginger. Sauté, stirring frequently, for 5 minutes, making sure they don't stick to the bottom of the pot.

3. Add the chicken broth, chicken, and salt. Cover, bring to a boil over high heat, then decrease the heat to medium and cook until the chicken is no longer pink inside, 4 to 5 minutes.

4. Remove from the heat. Add the zucchini noodles, enoki mushrooms, and scallions. Let rest for 5 minutes.

To assemble: Ladle the pho evenly among 4 containers or mason jars. I prefer to keep the fresh basil on the side, in a small resealable plastic bag, for instance, and add it at the last minute after reheating the soup.

Note: Store for up to 5 days in an airtight container in the refrigerator. Not suitable for freezing.

MOROCCAN CHICKEN *with* BUTTERNUT SQUASH RICE

My fragrant Moroccan chicken, served with Butternut Squash Rice, is sweet, savory, and spicy all at the same time. This aromatic North African dish pairs AIP-compliant spices, like cinnamon, ginger, and cloves, with black olives and peaches to create a meal that's a little like a traditional Moroccan tagine and a little like a South Asian curry—and it's utterly delicious!

Prep time:
10 minutes

Cook time:
26 minutes

Yield:
5 servings

1¼ pounds (568 g) boneless skinless chicken breasts

1 sweet potato (1 pound [454 g])

1 yellow onion (½ pound [227 g])

3 cloves garlic

2 tablespoons (30 ml) coconut oil, divided

1½ teaspoons sea salt, divided

¾ cup (180 ml) chicken Bone Broth (page 180)

1 cup (110 g) pitted black olives

½ teaspoon ground cinnamon

½ teaspoon ginger powder

⅛ teaspoon ground cloves

1 (15-ounce [420 g]) can sliced peaches, drained

1 recipe Butternut Squash Rice (page 176)

Minced fresh cilantro, for garnish

1. Cut the chicken into bite-size pieces. Peel and dice the sweet potato, chop the onion, and mince the garlic cloves.

2. Heat 1 tablespoon (15 ml) of the coconut oil in a large skillet over medium heat. When hot, add the chicken and ½ teaspoon of the salt, and mix well. Cover and cook until no longer pink, about 6 minutes. Transfer to a large bowl. Wipe the skillet clean and return to the heat.

3. Heat the remaining 1 tablespoon (15 ml) coconut oil. When hot, add the onion and garlic. Cover and cook, stirring occasionally, for 5 minutes. Add the sweet potatoes, chicken broth, olives, remaining 1 teaspoon salt, cinnamon, ginger, and cloves. Mix well, cover, and cook until the sweet potatoes are tender, about 10 minutes. Transfer to the large bowl containing the chicken, add the peaches, and mix well. Check the seasoning and adjust to taste.

4. Prepare the Butternut Squash Rice following the directions on page 176.

To assemble: Divide the ingredients evenly among 5 containers. Garnish with minced fresh cilantro.

Note: Store for up to 5 days in an airtight container in the refrigerator, or freeze for up to 4 months.

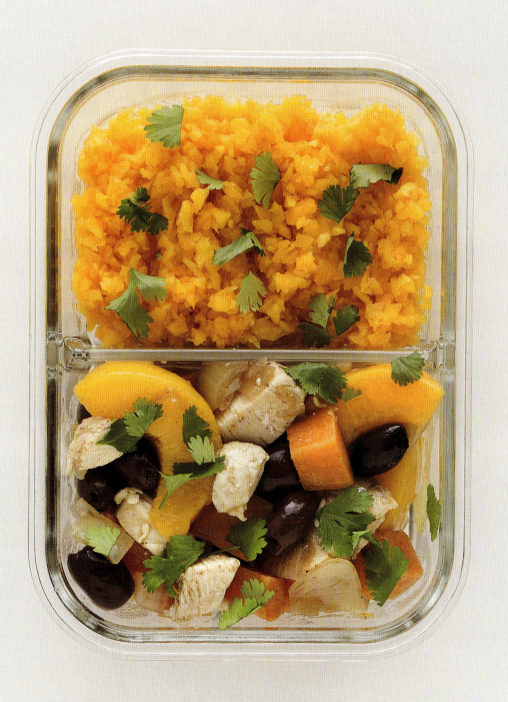

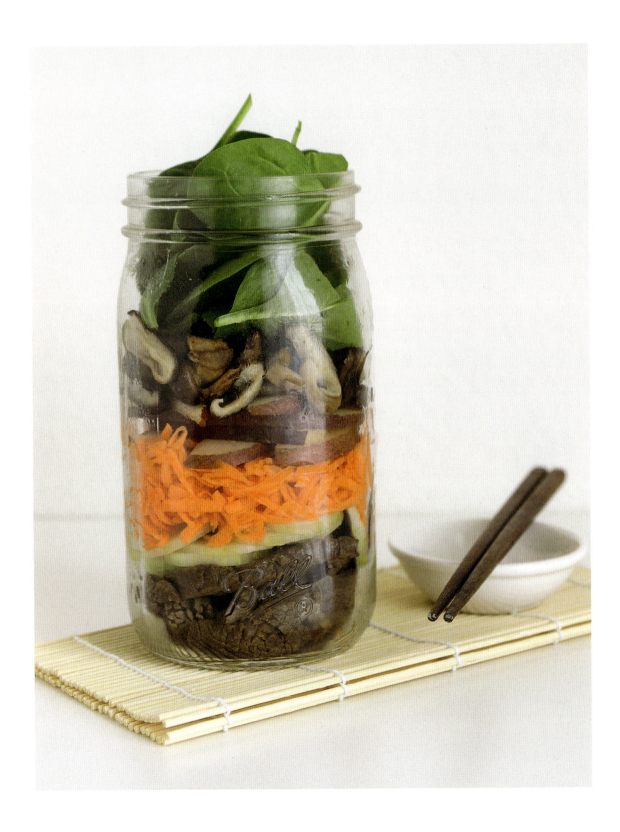

ASIAN STEAK SALAD

Marinated steak is the foundation of this vibrant Asian-inspired salad. The marinade needs time to infuse the meat with its rich flavor, so it's best to complete this step the day before and refrigerate overnight. Then you'll pair it with delicately flavored cucumber, pear, carrots, and spinach and top it with a gingery vinaigrette for a meal that's anything but ordinary.

Prep time:
15 minutes
Cook time:
13 minutes
Yield:
4 servings

FOR THE MARINADE:

Juice of 2 limes

3 tablespoons (45 ml) maple syrup

2 tablespoons (30 ml) coconut aminos

2 tablespoons (30 ml) fish sauce

1 (½-inch [1 cm]) piece ginger, peeled and grated

¾ pound (340 g) skirt steak

6 ounces (168 g) shiitake mushrooms

1 cucumber (10 ounces [280 g])

1 large pear

3 tablespoons (45 ml) coconut oil, divided

½ teaspoon sea salt

1 recipe Asian Dressing (page 178)

1⅓ cups (150 g) shredded carrot

½ pound (227 g) baby spinach

1. To make the marinade, whisk together the ingredients for the marinade and set aside. Slice the skirt steak into ⅓-inch (8 mm) strips and place in a large resealable plastic bag. Pour the marinade over the steak. Seal the bag and massage the steak, making sure all the pieces are well coated. Marinate in the refrigerator overnight (or for at least for 2 hours), turning the bag over a few times.

2. Slice the shiitake mushrooms. Peel and thinly slice the cucumber. Quarter, core, and thinly slice the pear.

3. Heat 2 tablespoons (30 ml) of the coconut oil in a large nonstick skillet over medium heat. When hot, add the mushrooms and salt, and cook, covered, until tender and lightly browned, about 8 minutes. (Adjust the temperature or add some liquid if the mushrooms stick to the bottom of the skillet.) Transfer to a plate and return the skillet to the heat.

4. Heat the remaining 1 tablespoon (15 ml) coconut oil in the skillet. When hot, add the steak strips with the marinade. Cover and cook until the meat is cooked through, 4 to 5 minutes. Transfer to a plate with a slotted spatula.

5. Make the Asian Dressing following the instructions on page 178.

To assemble: Divide the ingredients evenly among 4 containers or mason jars, starting with the steak strips at the bottom, followed by the cucumbers, carrots, pears, mushrooms, and spinach. I prefer to keep the dressing on the side, in a small container, and add it at the last minute before serving. You can also add the dressing at the very bottom of the jar before you add the other ingredients and shake well before serving.

Note: Store for up to 5 days in an airtight container in the refrigerator. Not suitable for freezing.

THAI CURRY MEATBALLS

I used to love a good curry before my AIP days, so I've worked hard to recreate a rich, creamy, and spicy curry—and here it is! The secret ingredients that make this AIP-friendly curry sauce so phenomenal? Sweet potato and coconut milk for the base, then fresh garlic, fresh ginger, basil, and lime juice for lots of kick!

Prep time:
20 minutes
Cook time:
36 minutes
Yield:
4 servings

FOR THE MEATBALLS:

1 pound (454 g) ground chicken

1 carrot (6 ounces [168 g]), shredded

1 zucchini (6 ounces [168 g]), shredded

1 tablespoon (4 g) minced fresh basil

1 teaspoon sea salt

1 tablespoon (15 ml) coconut oil

FOR THE CURRY SAUCE:

1 sweet potato (1 pound [454 g]), peeled and diced

1 (14-ounce [392 ml]) can full-fat coconut milk

2 tablespoons (30 ml) coconut oil

1 onion (½ pound [227 g]), minced

3 large cloves garlic, minced

1 (1½-inch [3.8 cm]) knob fresh ginger, peeled and grated

1 tablespoon (4 g) minced fresh basil

Juice of ½ lime

1½ teaspoons sea salt

1 recipe Cauliflower Rice (page 177)

1. To make the meatballs, combine the ground chicken, carrot, zucchini, basil, and salt in a bowl and mix thoroughly using your hands. Form into 8 meatballs. Heat the coconut oil in a large skillet over medium heat. When hot, add the meatballs and cook until no longer pink inside, about 15 minutes, turning them over halfway through. When done, transfer to a plate.

2. To make the curry sauce, add the sweet potatoes to a medium saucepan and cover with water. Bring to a boil over high heat, then decrease the heat to medium and cook, covered, until tender, about 12 minutes. When done, drain the water and transfer the sweet potatoes to a food processor equipped with an S-blade. Add the coconut milk and blend until smooth, about 30 seconds. Set aside.

3. Heat the coconut oil in a saucepan over medium-high heat. When hot, add the onions and cook, stirring frequently, until they start to brown, about 8 minutes. (If the onions stick to the bottom of the pan, add more oil or reduce the heat.)

4. Decrease the heat to low; add the garlic, ginger, and basil; and sauté for 1 minute while stirring. Add the sweet potato and coconut mixture, lime juice, and salt, and mix well. Check the seasoning and adjust to taste.

5. Make the Cauliflower Rice following the directions on page 177.

To assemble: Divide the ingredients evenly among 4 containers, starting with a layer of cauliflower rice at the bottom, followed by the meatballs and a generous serving of curry sauce on top.

Note: Store for up to 5 days in an airtight container in the refrigerator, or freeze for up to 4 months.

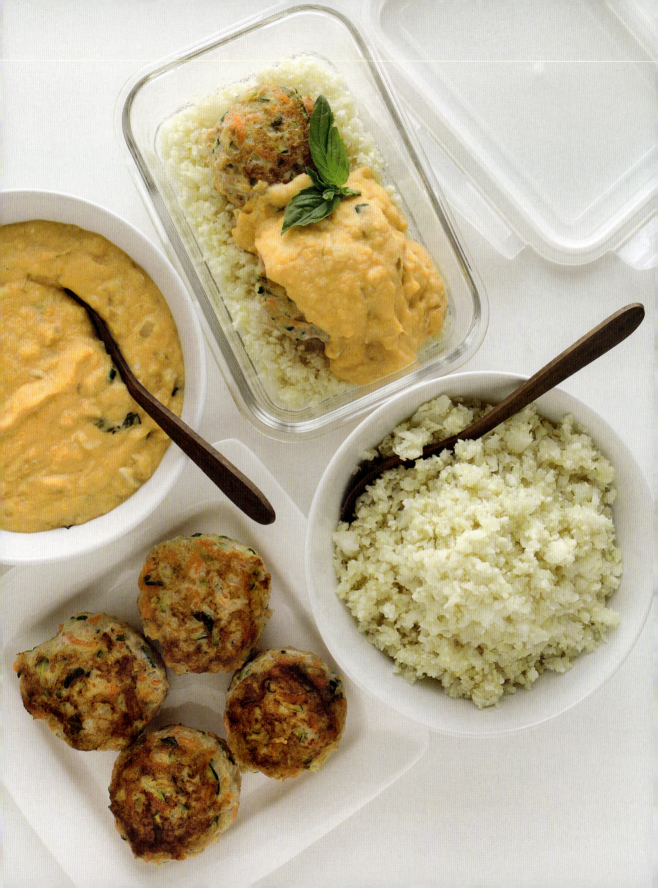

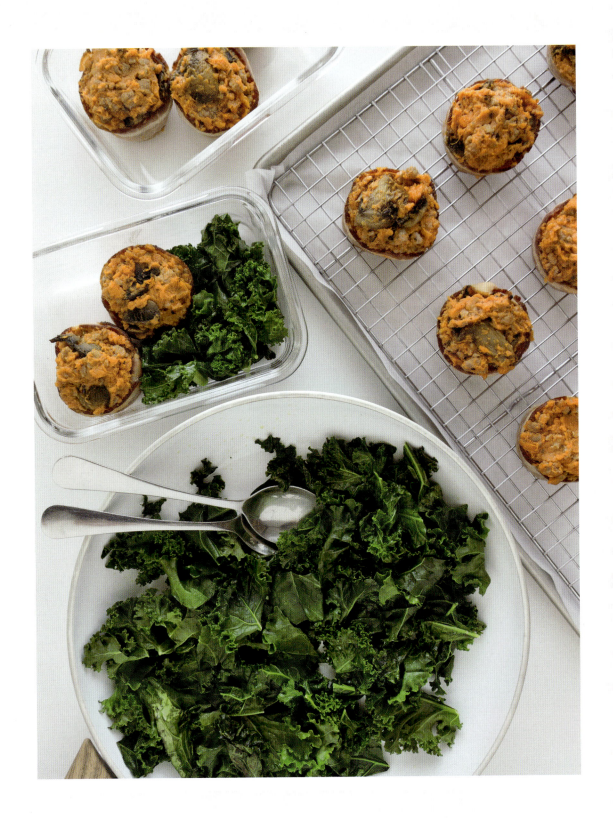

Chapter 11
SUPERBOWL MEAL PLAN

G et ready to party all week with the Superbowl Meal Plan! This fun menu combines crowd-friendly favorites with plenty of nutritious, fiber-rich vegetables to keep you cheering all week long.

While the recipes in this menu are a little on the labor-intensive side, the whole batch-cooking session and cleanup still shouldn't take you more than half a day at the most (unless you're watching the game at the same time, of course!).

Shepherd's Pie Bacon Cups make for a convenient breakfast option on those mornings when time is tight. They combine slow carbs (for sustained energy) with lots of vegetables and turkey (an easy-to-digest protein), all neatly wrapped in yummy bacon cups!

Next, there's a spin on the traditional loaded sweet potatoes. My **Broccoli and Cheese Stuffed Sweet Potatoes** feature a dairy-free cheese sauce that is incredibly versatile, easy to whip up, and makes a great topping for lots of other dishes, too.

This week's snack is a game-day classic: **Teriyaki Chicken Wings** are on the menu! Cutlery is optional here, but you'll definitely want to have a few extra napkins (or moist towelettes) on hand for easy cleanup. If you're preparing this dish for a party, try doubling the Teriyaki Sauce and serving half of it on the side so that your guests can double-dip.

The **Cheeseburger Casserole** is all kinds of yummy, and no one will know—or care—that it's dairy-free. With lots of vegetables, beef, and bacon, plus a secret ingredient, this dairy-free casserole will definitely make it to the playoffs!

Finally, I've lined up another fun-to-eat finger food to round off your week. Paired with fresh-cut vegetables and a succulent no-cook BBQ sauce, my **BBQ Party Meatballs** will disappear at lightning speed the minute you serve them to a group.

Kitchen note: Don't forget to marinate the **Teriyaki Chicken Wings** the day before your batch-cooking session (see directions on page 141), and make sure you have ⅓ cup (80 ml) of chicken Bone Broth ready.

	BREAKFAST	LUNCH	DINNER	SNACK
DAY 1	Shepherd's Pie Bacon Cups	Broccoli and Cheese Stuffed Sweet Potatoes	Cheeseburger Casserole	Teriyaki Chicken Wings
DAY 2	Shepherd's Pie Bacon Cups	BBQ Party Meatballs	Broccoli and Cheese Stuffed Sweet Potatoes	Teriyaki Chicken Wings
DAY 3	Cheeseburger Casserole	Broccoli and Cheese Stuffed Sweet Potatoes	BBQ Party Meatballs	Teriyaki Chicken Wings
DAY 4	Shepherd's Pie Bacon Cups	BBQ Party Meatballs	Cheeseburger Casserole	Teriyaki Chicken Wings
DAY 5	Shepherd's Pie Bacon Cups	Broccoli and Cheese Stuffed Sweet Potatoes	Cheeseburger Casserole	Teriyaki Chicken Wings

EXTRA SERVINGS: 1 BBQ Party Meatballs

Shopping List

PRODUCE

2 limes

3 scallions

1 yellow onion (½ pound [227 g])

10 ounces (280 g) mushrooms

¾ pound (340 g) carrots

1 bunch celery (¾ pound [340 g])

2 (8-ounce [227 g]) bunches kale

1¼ pounds (568 g) white sweet potatoes

1½ pounds (680 g) broccoli florets

3 pounds (1362 g) cauliflower florets

7 (10-ounce [280 g]) sweet potatoes

MEAT/SEAFOOD

⅓ cup (80 ml) chicken Bone Broth (page 180)

1 pound (454 g) ground pork

12 slices thick-cut bacon (¾ pound [340 g]) + ¾ pound (340 g) thick-cut bacon

2 pounds (908 g) chicken wings

2¼ pounds (1 kg) ground beef

HERBS AND SPICES

1¼ teaspoons onion powder

1½ teaspoons ginger powder

2¾ teaspoons garlic powder

1 tablespoon (2 g) dried sage

PANTRY ITEMS

1 tablespoon (8 g) arrowroot starch

2 tablespoons (16 g) coconut flour

2 tablespoons (30 ml) maple syrup

2½ tablespoons (50 g) blackstrap molasses

¼ cup (60 ml) apple cider vinegar

½ cup + ⅓ cup (35 g + 25 g) nutritional yeast

1 cup + 1 tablespoon (235 ml + 15 ml) coconut aminos

1½ cups (240 g) unsweetened applesauce

OTHER

Coconut oil

Extra-virgin olive oil

Sea salt

Equipment and Tools

15 containers for your meals + 5 containers for snacks (see pages 32 to 33)

12-cup nonstick muffin pan

2 large rimmed baking sheets (12 x 17 inches [30.5 x 43 cm])

chef's knife, paring knife

containers

cutting board

high-speed blender

large skillet (at least 11 inches [28 cm] wide)

measuring cups and spoons

mixing bowl

potato masher (or food processor with S-blade)

pots and pans

slotted spatula

vegetable peeler

whisk

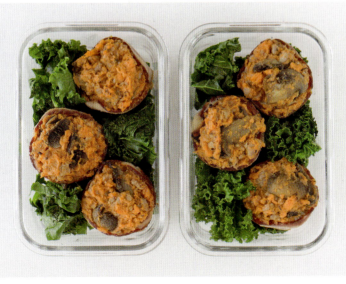

Batch-Cooking Directions

1. Reminder: *The morning before*, defrost the meat if frozen. *The day before*, complete steps 1 and 2 of the **Teriyaki Chicken Wings** (page 141). Make sure you have ⅓ cup (80 ml) of chicken **Bone Broth** (page 180) on hand. Prepare your containers.

2. The day of your batch-cooking session, preheat the oven to 400°F (200°C or gas mark 6). Place a rack in the middle of the oven, and one at the bottom (second to the last slot).

3. Complete steps 1 and 2 of the **Shepherd's Pie Bacon Cups** (page 139) as well as steps 1 and 2 of the **Broccoli and Cheese Stuffed Sweet Potatoes** (page 142). Place all the sweet potatoes on the same baking sheet and bake on the middle rack in the oven. Set a timer for 60 minutes.

4. Complete steps 3 through 5 of the **Teriyaki Chicken Wings** (page 141), and bake on the bottom rack in the oven. Set a timer for 30 minutes and remember to flip the wings halfway through.

5. While the sweet potatoes and chicken wings are in the oven, complete steps 3 through 6 of the **Shepherd's Pie Bacon Cups** (page 139).

6. When the timer goes off for the sweet potatoes, complete steps 7 through 9 of the **Shepherd's Pie Bacon Cups** (page 139) and assemble. Also assemble the **Teriyaki Chicken Wings** (page 141).

7. Complete steps 3 through 5 of the **Broccoli and Cheese Stuffed Sweet Potatoes** (page 142) and assemble.

8. Complete the **Cheeseburger Casserole** (page 145), steps 1 through 5, and assemble.

9. Complete the **BBQ Party Meatballs** (page 146), steps 1 through 5, and assemble.

SHEPHERD'S PIE BACON CUPS

Put anything into a bacon cup and it's instantly more fun to eat, right? Paired with wilted kale for a balanced meal, these miniature sweet potato-based shepherd's pies are an especially good breakfast option, delivering sustained energy and a whole lot of flavor!

Prep time:
20 minutes
Cook time:
1 hour
Yield:
4 to 6 servings

3 (10-ounce [280 g]) sweet potatoes

12 slices bacon, thick cut (¾ pound [340 g])

10 ounces (280 g) mushrooms, sliced

4 tablespoons (60 ml) olive oil, divided

1 tablespoon (2 g) dried sage

1½ teaspoons sea salt, divided, plus more as needed

1 pound (454 g) ground pork

2 (½-pound [227 g]) bunches kale, destemmed and chopped

1. Preheat the oven to 400°F (200°C or gas mark 6) and place the rack in the middle. Line a rimmed baking sheet with parchment paper.

2. Poke holes in the sweet potatoes, then place on the baking sheet. Bake for 50 to 60 minutes or until a paring knife inserted in the middle of the sweet potatoes easily goes all the way through.

3. Line each hole of a 12-cup nonstick muffin pan with a slice of bacon, forming a cup.

4. Heat 2 tablespoons (30 ml) of the olive oil in a large skillet over medium heat. When hot, add the mushrooms, dried sage, and ¾ teaspoon of the salt. Mix well, cover, and cook until tender, about 10 minutes. Transfer to a large mixing bowl.

5. Heat 1 tablespoon (15 ml) of the olive oil in the skillet over medium heat. When hot, add the ground pork and remaining salt. Cook until no longer pink, about 6 minutes. Use a slotted spatula to transfer to the mixing bowl with the mushrooms. Wipe the skillet clean.

6. Heat the remaining olive oil in the skillet over medium heat. When hot, add the kale, cover, and cook until wilted, about 3 minutes. Season to taste with salt.

7. When the sweet potatoes are cool, peel and mash them.

8. Combine the sweet potato with the mushrooms and pork. Mix well. Adjust the salt to taste.

9. Spoon the mixture into the bacon cups and bake for 20 minutes until the bacon is fully cooked.

To assemble: Divide the sweet potato muffins and kale evenly among 4 or 6 containers.

Note: Store for up to 5 days in an airtight container in the refrigerator, or freeze for up to 4 months.

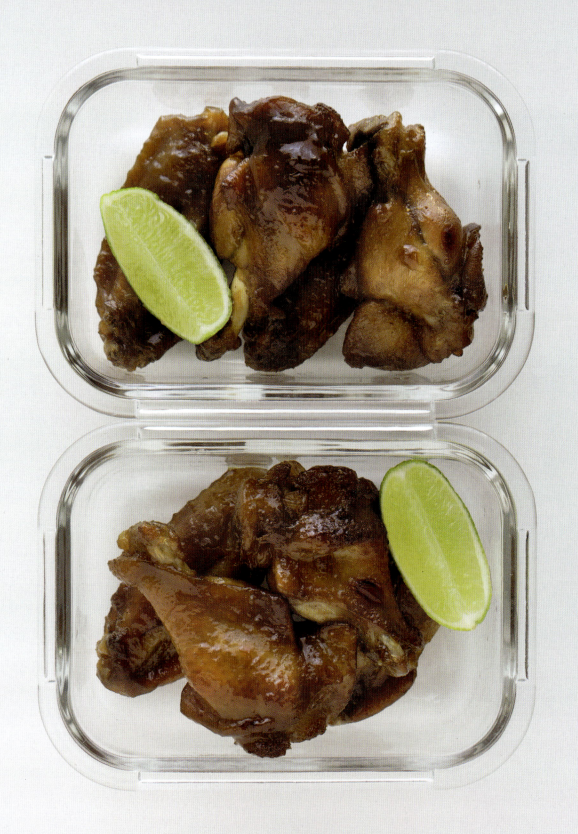

TERIYAKI CHICKEN WINGS

These sticky chicken wings are delicious any time of day and make for a perfect snack, hot or cold. If you purchased whole chicken wings, cut and save the wing tips to make chicken Bone Broth (page 180), then cut once more at the joint between the flap and the drumette. Use a sharp paring knife for this, or even a chef's knife.

Prep time:
10 minutes +
marinating time
Cook time:
30 minutes
Yield:
5 servings

1 recipe Teriyaki Sauce (page 186)

20 chicken wing pieces (about 2 pounds [908 g])

2 limes, cut into wedges

1. The day before, mix all the ingredients for the Teriyaki Sauce (page 186), except the arrowroot flour, in a small bowl.

2. Add the chicken wings to a large resealable plastic bag and pour the teriyaki mixture over. Seal the bag and massage, making sure all the wings are well coated. Marinate in the refrigerator overnight (or for at least 2 hours), turning the bag over a few times.

3. Preheat the oven to 400°F (200°C or gas mark 6) and place the rack in the middle (or at the bottom, second-to-the-last slot, if you are following the batch-cooking directions). Line a rimmed baking sheet or broiler pan with aluminum foil.

4. Remove the wings from the refrigerator, open the plastic bag, and sprinkle 1½ tablespoons (12 g) arrowroot flour over the wings. Reseal the bag and massage thoroughly.

5. Transfer the wings to the baking sheet, including the leftover marinade, and bake in the oven for about 30 minutes, until nicely brown, flipping the wings over halfway through.

To assemble: Divide the chicken wings evenly among 5 glass containers, adding a lime wedge in each container for squeezing and drizzling right before eating.

Note: Store for up to 5 days in an airtight container in the refrigerator, or freeze for up to 4 months. (If freezing, do not add the lime wedge until you are ready to serve.)

BROCCOLI *and* CHEESE STUFFED SWEET POTATOES

Broccoli and cheese is the perfect marriage of saintly and sinful—except this healthy recipe is completely guilt-free! It's packed with antioxidants, too. Pro tip: Try to select sweet potatoes of the same size so that they cook evenly in the oven. And when you're ready to assemble, you may have to scoop out some of the sweet potato flesh to make room for the broccoli and the luscious dairy-free cheese sauce!

Prep time:
15 minutes
Cook time:
60 minutes
Yield:
4 servings

4 (10-ounce [280 g]) sweet potatoes
¾ pound (340 g) broccoli florets
1 recipe Dairy-Free Cheese Sauce
(page 182)
Sea salt

1. Preheat the oven to 400°F (200°C or gas mark 6) and place the rack in the middle. Line a rimmed baking sheet with parchment paper.

2. Poke holes in the sweet potatoes a few times with a fork, then line them up on the baking sheet. Bake in the oven until tender and cooked through, 50 to 60 minutes. To check whether the sweet potatoes are cooked through, insert a paring knife in the middle. The flesh should feel soft and tender all the way through.

3. Meanwhile, add the broccoli florets to a saucepan and cover with water. Bring to a boil over high heat, then decrease the heat to medium and cook until crisp-tender, about 8 minutes. Drain and set aside.

4. Prepare the Dairy-Free Cheese Sauce, following the directions on page 182.

5. When the sweet potatoes are done, transfer to a plate to cool slightly, then cut a slit lengthwise in each, allowing space for stuffing with the broccoli (you may have to scoop out some sweet potato flesh), and season with salt to taste.

To assemble: You can assemble this dish in two ways. You can stuff each sweet potato with broccoli (don't forget to season with salt to taste as well) and cheese sauce, then wrap them in aluminum foil. Or you can cut each sweet potato in half lengthwise and place each half cut-face up at the bottom of the containers. Follow with a layer of broccoli on top (season with salt to taste) and a serving of cheese sauce.

Note: Store for up to 5 days in an airtight container in the refrigerator, or freeze for up to 4 months.

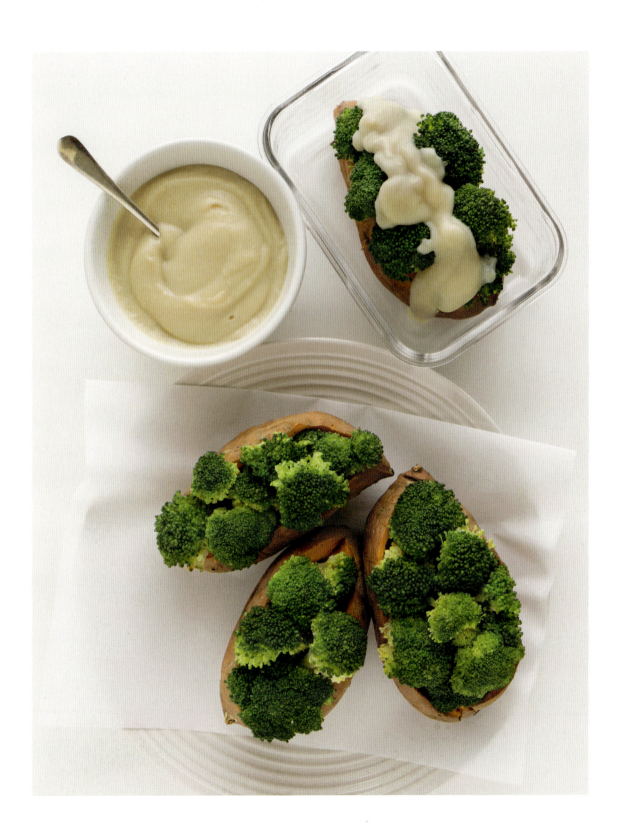

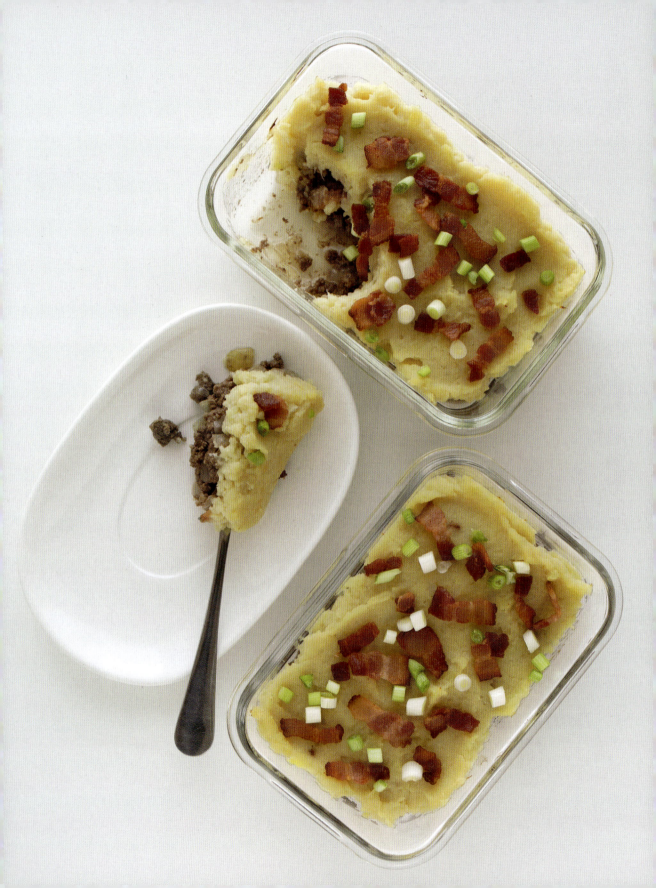

CHEESEBURGER CASSEROLE

Cheese isn't an AIP-compliant ingredient. But who can live without its rich, savory taste? Not me! Never fear: This is where an ancient Egyptian superfood called nutritional yeast comes to the rescue, supplying plenty of umami flavor. It plays a key role in this good-for-you casserole—which, by the way, is much faster to make than the traditional version because there are no eggs, so there's no need for a second bake.

Prep time:
15 minutes
Cook time:
45 minutes
Yield:
4 servings

1¼ pounds (568 g) white sweet potatoes

1¼ pounds (568 g) cauliflower florets

¾ pound (340 g) bacon

1 yellow onion (½ pound [227 g])

3 scallions

⅓ cup (25 g) nutritional yeast

1½ teaspoons sea salt, divided

1 pound (454 g) ground beef

1. Peel and dice the sweet potatoes. Add the sweet potatoes and cauliflower florets to a saucepan and cover with water. Cover with a lid, bring to a boil over high heat, then decrease the heat to medium and cook until tender, about 20 minutes.

2. While the vegetables are cooking, cut the bacon into ¼-inch (6 mm) strips, dice the onion, and slice the scallions.

3. When the vegetables are done, drain them well. Then, using a potato masher, mash the vegetables until you obtain a puree (you may also do this in a food processor equipped with an S-blade). Stir in the nutritional yeast and ¾ teaspoon of the salt. Check the seasoning and adjust to taste. Set aside.

4. In a large skillet over medium heat, cook the bacon until golden brown, 8 to 10 minutes. Using a slotted spatula, transfer the bacon to a paper towel–lined plate, reserving the bacon fat in the skillet (you may have to add more cooking oil if the bacon didn't render enough fat).

5. Add the onions and cook until tender, about 8 minutes. Add the ground beef and the remaining ¾ teaspoon salt and cook for another 8 minutes, until browned. Add the bacon back to the skillet (reserving some for garnish) and mix well.

To assemble: Using a slotted spatula, divide the meat mixture evenly among 4 glass containers. Top each with a layer of puree and garnish with crumbled bacon and sliced scallion.

Note: Store for up to 5 days in an airtight container in the refrigerator, or freeze for up to 4 months.

BBQ PARTY MEATBALLS

So quick and easy to pull together and smothered in thick, rich, no-cook BBQ sauce, these little meatballs make great party food—especially when last-minute guests turn up! Serve them with raw vegetables for a balanced meal. (Save additional time by buying ready-cut veggies at the store.)

Prep time:
20 minutes
Cook time:
10 minutes
Yield:
4 servings

1 pound (454 g) ground beef

2 tablespoons (16 g) coconut flour

1 tablespoon (15 ml) coconut aminos

¾ teaspoon sea salt

¼ teaspoon garlic powder

¼ teaspoon onion powder

1 recipe No-Cook BBQ Sauce
    (page 184)

¾ pound (340 g) carrots

1 small bunch celery (¾ pound
    [227 g])

¾ pound (340 g) broccoli florets

¾ pound (340 g) cauliflower florets

1. Combine the ground beef, coconut flour, coconut aminos, salt, garlic powder, and onion powder in a large bowl. Mix thoroughly using your hands.

2. Scooping out 1 tablespoon (15 g)-size portion of the meat mixture at a time, form into 24 meatballs, then transfer them to a large skillet.

3. Prepare the No-Cook BBQ Sauce following the directions on page 184 and pour the sauce over the meatballs.

4. Cover and cook the meatballs over medium heat until they are no longer pink inside, about 10 minutes.

5. Meanwhile, peel and cut the carrots into sticks. Cut the celery into sticks as well.

To assemble: Serve the raw vegetables alongside the meatballs. I like to keep the ingredients separate in this meal, so I prefer to use containers with built-in compartments, storing the meatballs on one side and the vegetables on the other. If you don't have such containers, I suggest using two separate containers—or use a resealable plastic bag for the veggies.

Note: Store for up to 5 days in an airtight container in the refrigerator, or freeze for up to 4 months and cut up the vegetables when ready to serve.

If you like, you can serve this meal with an extra side of leafy greens and Tzatziki Dressing (page 188) for dipping the veggies!

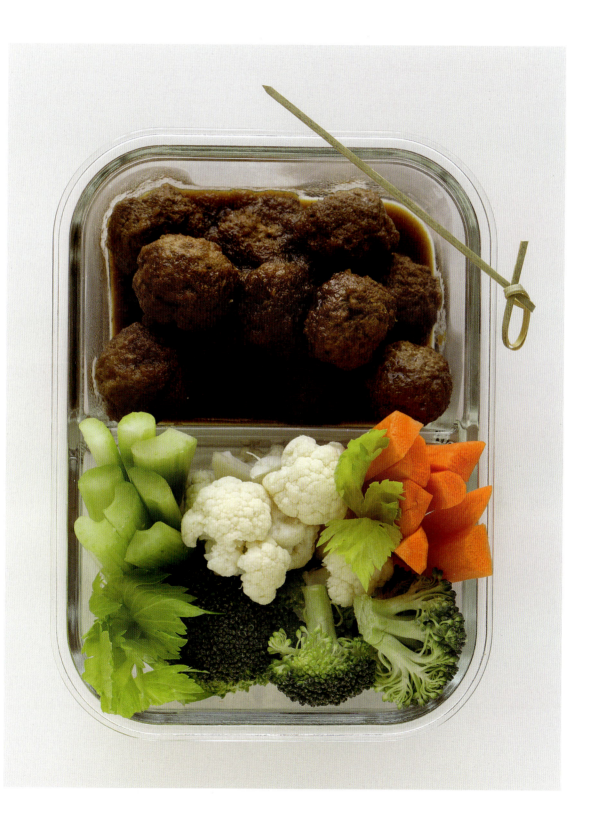

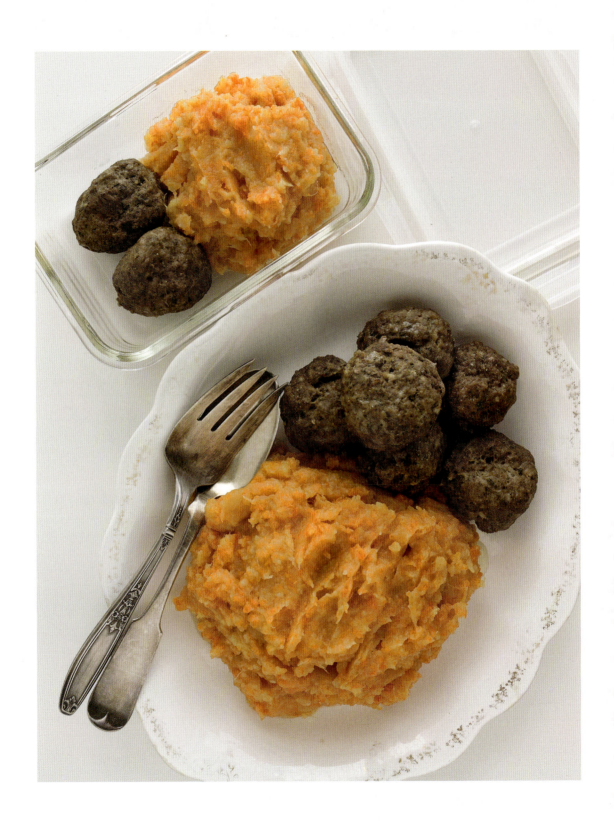

Chapter 12
ONE-POT MEAL PLAN

When life gets busy, it's hard enough to find time to cook healthy, AIP-compliant meals, never mind the kitchen cleanup afterward. That's why each meal on your menu this week fits in a single cooking vessel, whether that's a skillet, a stockpot, a pressure cooker, or an Instant Pot: There's way less washing up to do after your batch-cooking session! And as usual, they're all simple, wholesome meals that are easy to reheat and enjoy.

First on the menu is a household classic: **Meatballs and Veggie Mash**. This gentle, comforting meal is ready in less than half an hour from start to finish—and you get to sit back and relax while your pressure cooker or Instant Pot does all the work for you. Genius!

Next, my **Turmeric Chicken Soup** is made in a large stockpot on the stovetop. The gut-healing benefits of chicken bone broth plus the anti-inflammatory properties of turmeric mean that this deceptively simple soup is actually a nutritional powerhouse!

Then you'll make the **Garlic Beef Stew** in your pressure cooker or Instant Pot: It's both restorative and fragrant, relying on AIP-approved herbs and spices such as garlic, sage, thyme, and bay leaf for its rich, autumnal flavor.

How about a lush **Blueberry Mousse** for a snack? Lightly sweet and full of fruit, it requires only minimal preparation (and no cooking whatsoever)!

Last comes one of my favorites: my **Chicken Fried Rice Skillet**. If you've been missing Chinese takeout, you'll be able to scratch the itch with this single-skillet wonder. How? Cauliflower Rice makes this dish AIP compliant, while liquid coconut aminos is used in lieu of soy sauce.

Kitchen note: Make sure you have 2 cups (480 ml) of beef Bone Broth and 2 quarts + ¾ cup (2 L + 180 ml) of chicken Bone Broth on hand.

	BREAKFAST	LUNCH	DINNER	SNACK
DAY 1	Turmeric Chicken Soup	Meatballs and Veggie Mash	Chicken Fried Rice Skillet	Blueberry Mousse
DAY 2	Garlic Beef Stew	Turmeric Chicken Soup	Meatballs and Veggie Mash	Blueberry Mousse
DAY 3	Chicken Fried Rice Skillet	Garlic Beef Stew	Turmeric Chicken Soup	Blueberry Mousse
DAY 4	Meatballs and Veggie Mash	Chicken Fried Rice Skillet	Garlic Beef Stew	Blueberry Mousse
DAY 5	Turmeric Chicken Soup	Meatballs and Veggie Mash	Chicken Fried Rice Skillet	Blueberry Mousse

EXTRA SERVINGS: 1 Garlic Beef Stew + 1 Turmeric Chicken Soup

Shopping List

PRODUCE

1 leek (¾ pound [340 g])

2 cups (300 g) frozen blueberries

1 pound (454 g) cauliflower florets

1 pound (454 g) celery ribs

1 pound (454 g) sweet potatoes

2 yellow onions (½ pound + ¾ pound [227 g + 340 g])

1¼ pounds (568 g) turnips

2 pounds (908 g) white sweet potatoes

3¼ pounds (1476 g) carrots

4 scallions

5 cloves garlic

MEAT/SEAFOOD

2 cups (480 ml) beef Bone Broth (page 180)

½ pound (227 g) ground pork

¾ pound (340 g) ground beef

1½ pounds (680 g) beef stew meat

2¼ pounds (1 kg) boneless skinless chicken breasts

2 quarts + ¾ cup (2 L + 180 ml) chicken Bone Broth (page 180)

HERBS AND SPICES

1 bay leaf

½ teaspoon dried thyme

1 teaspoon garlic powder

1 teaspoon ginger powder

1½ teaspoons ground turmeric

1 tablespoon (2 g) dried parsley

1 tablespoon (2 g) dried sage

PANTRY ITEMS

1 tablespoon (8 g) coconut flour

1½ tablespoons (12 g) gelatin powder

2 tablespoons (30 ml) maple syrup

¾ cup + 1 tablespoon (180 ml + 15 ml) coconut
aminos

1 (14-ounce [392 ml]) can + 1 cup (240 ml)
full-fat coconut milk

OTHER

Coconut oil

Extra-virgin olive oil

Sea salt

Equipment and Tools

15 containers for your meals + 5 containers for
snacks (see pages 32–33)

aluminum foil

chef's knife

cutting board

electric pressure cooker with trivet
(or Instant Pot)

food processor with S-blade

ladle

large skillet (at least 11 inches [28 cm] wide)

measuring cups and spoons

mixing bowls

potato masher

slotted spatula

stockpot

vegetable peeler

Batch-Cooking Directions

1. Reminder: *The morning before*, defrost the meat if frozen. Make sure you have 2 cups (480 ml) of beef **Bone Broth** (page 180) and 2 quarts + ¾ cup (2 L + 180 ml) of chicken **Bone Broth** (page 180) on hand. Prepare your containers.

2. Start your batch-cooking session with the **Meatballs and Veggie Mash** (page 153). Complete steps 1 through 3 and start cooking in your Instant Pot.

3. Meanwhile, complete the **Turmeric Chicken Soup** (page 155), steps 1 and 2, and set a timer for 20 minutes.

4. When the Instant Pot beeps, complete steps 4 and 5 of the **Meatballs and Veggie Mash** (page 153), and assemble. When the timer goes off for the soup, assemble.

5. Next, complete the **Garlic Beef Stew** (page 156), steps 1 through 4.

6. While you are waiting for the Instant Pot to beep, complete the **Blueberry Mousse** (page 159), steps 1 through 3, and assemble.

7. When the Instant Pot beeps, complete step 5 of the **Garlic Beef Stew** (page 156), and assemble.

8. Finish your batch-cooking session with the **Chicken Fried Rice Skillet** (page 160), steps 1 through 5, and assemble.

(INSTANT POT) MEATBALLS *and* VEGGIE MASH

If you're craving something comforting and nutritious that's ready in minutes but don't feel like dealing with a ton of prep and cleanup, you'll thank me for this quick, AIP-compliant fix. These protein-rich meatballs paired with a satisfying veggie mash come to life in your Instant Pot or pressure cooker while you chill out on the couch.

Prep time:
10 minutes
Cook time:
20 minutes
Yield:
4 servings

FOR THE MASH:

2 pounds (908 g) white sweet potatoes

1 pound (454 g) carrots

¾ cup (180 ml) coconut milk

1 tablespoon (15 ml) coconut aminos

¾ teaspoon sea salt

FOR THE MEATBALLS:

¾ pound (340 g) ground beef

½ pound (227 g) ground pork

2 tablespoons (30 ml) coconut aminos

1 tablespoon (8 g) coconut flour

1 tablespoon (2 g) dried parsley

1 teaspoon sea salt

1. To make the mash, peel the sweet potatoes and carrots, then chop into 2-inch (5 cm) pieces (they will overcook if you cut them any smaller). Place them at the bottom of the Instant Pot, add the coconut milk, and place the trivet on top.

2. To make the meatballs, in a large bowl, use your hands to combine the beef, pork, coconut aminos, coconut flour, parsley, and salt. Form 8 balls of equal size, then wrap the meatballs in a piece of aluminum foil and place them on top of the trivet.

3. Close the lid of the Instant Pot, turn the pressure valve to the SEALING position, press MANUAL, and adjust the time to 20 minutes using the +/- buttons.

4. When the Instant Pot beeps, quick-release the pressure. Open the lid and carefully remove the wrapped meatballs and the trivet. When the meatballs are cool enough to handle, unwrap.

5. Use a potato masher to mash the vegetables. Stir in the coconut aminos and salt.

STOVETOP DIRECTIONS

1. Place the sweet potatoes and carrots in a large saucepan and cover with water. Cook over medium heat until tender, about 15 minutes. Drain well, then mash with a potato masher. Stir in the coconut milk, coconut aminos, and salt. Mix well.

2. Prepare the meatballs as described in step 2 above (skipping the aluminum foil). Heat 1 tablespoon (15 ml) of olive oil in a large skillet over medium heat. When hot, add the meatballs and cook until golden and no longer pink inside, 12 to 15 minutes.

To assemble: Divide the ingredients evenly among 4 containers.

Note: Store for up to 5 days in an airtight container in the refrigerator, or freeze for up to 4 months.

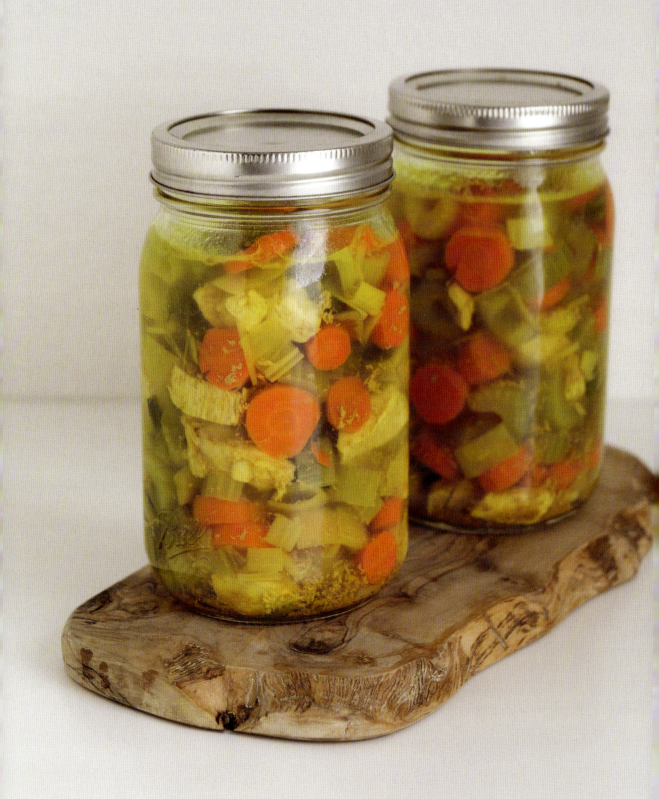

(STOCKPOT) TURMERIC CHICKEN SOUP

There's no better winter pick-me-up than this cheerful, bright-yellow soup. Pop a handful of basic ingredients into your stockpot or electric pressure cooker and in 20 minutes you'll be rewarded with a veggie-laden, collagen-rich, cockles-of-your-heart-warming meal. You're welcome!

Prep time:
10 minutes
Cook time:
20 minutes
Yield:
5 (16-ounce [454 g]) servings

1¼ pounds (568 g) boneless skinless chicken breasts

1 pound (454 g) carrots

1 pound (454 g) celery ribs

1 leek (¾ pound [340 g])

1 tablespoon (15 ml) extra-virgin olive oil

2 teaspoons sea salt

1½ teaspoons ground turmeric

2 quarts (2 L) chicken Bone Broth (page 180)

1. Dice the chicken breasts into bite-size pieces. Peel and slice the carrots. Slice the celery and the leek.

2. Add all the ingredients to the stockpot. Cover and bring to a boil over high heat, then decrease the heat to medium and cook until the vegetables are tender, 15 to 20 minutes. Check the seasoning and adjust to taste.

PRESSURE COOKER DIRECTIONS

1. Add all the ingredients to the pot of your electric pressure cooker (or Instant Pot). Close the lid, making sure the valve is in the SEALING position. Press MANUAL and adjust the time to 20 minutes using the +/- button. When the Instant Pot beeps, quick-release the pressure. Check the seasoning and adjust to taste.

To assemble: Divide the soup evenly among 5 containers or glass jars.

Note: Store for up to 5 days in an airtight container in the refrigerator, or freeze for up to 4 months.

(INSTANT POT) GARLIC BEEF STEW

Surrounded by fiber-rich root vegetables and bone broth (which combats inflammation and promotes a healthy immune system, thanks to the vital amino acids it contains), this meaty stew will sustain you through even the wettest, wildest winter days. And it freezes especially well!

Prep time:
10 minutes
Cook time:
38 minutes
Yield:
4 servings

1¼ pounds (568 g) turnips

1 pound (454 g) sweet potatoes

½ pound (227 g) carrots

1 yellow onion (¾ pound [340 g])

5 cloves garlic

3 tablespoons (45 ml) coconut oil, divided

1½ pounds (680 g) beef stew meat

2 cups (480 ml) beef Bone Broth (page 180)

1 tablespoon (2 g) dried sage

2 teaspoons sea salt, divided

½ teaspoon dried thyme

1 bay leaf

1. Dice the turnips. Peel and dice the sweet potatoes and slice the carrots. Chop the onion. Thinly slice the garlic cloves.

2. Press the SAUTÉ function on your Instant Pot and ADJUST the temperature to high. Heat 2 tablespoons (30 ml) of the coconut oil in the pot. When hot, add the onions and garlic, and cook, stirring frequently, for 5 minutes. Transfer to a plate.

3. Heat the remaining 1 tablespoon (15 ml) coconut oil in the pot. When hot, add the meat and brown on all sides, 2 to 3 minutes. You may have to do this in two batches.

4. Press CANCEL. Return the onions and garlic to the pot, plus the bone broth, sage, 1 teaspoon of the salt, thyme, and bay leaf. Close the lid, making sure the valve is in the SEALING position. Press MANUAL and adjust the time to 18 minutes using the +/- button.

5. When the Instant Pot beeps, quick-release the pressure. Open the lid and add the turnips, sweet potatoes, carrots, and remaining 1 teaspoon salt. Close the lid and the valve, press MANUAL, and adjust the time to 8 minutes using the +/- button. When the Instant Pot beeps, quick-release the pressure again. Discard the bay leaf. Check the seasoning and adjust to taste.

STOVETOP DIRECTIONS

1. Heat 2 tablespoons (30 ml) of the coconut oil in a stockpot over medium heat. When hot, add the meat and brown on all sides. You may have to do this in two batches.

2. Add the broth, sage, salt, thyme, and bay leaf. Cover and bring to a boil over high heat, then decrease the heat to medium-low and simmer for 1 hour.

3. Add the turnips, sweet potatoes, carrots, onions, and garlic, and continue to cook for 50 minutes. When done, discard the bay leaf and adjust the seasoning to taste.

To assemble: Divide the stew evenly among 4 containers.

Note: Store for up to 5 days in an airtight container in the refrigerator, or freeze for up to 4 months.

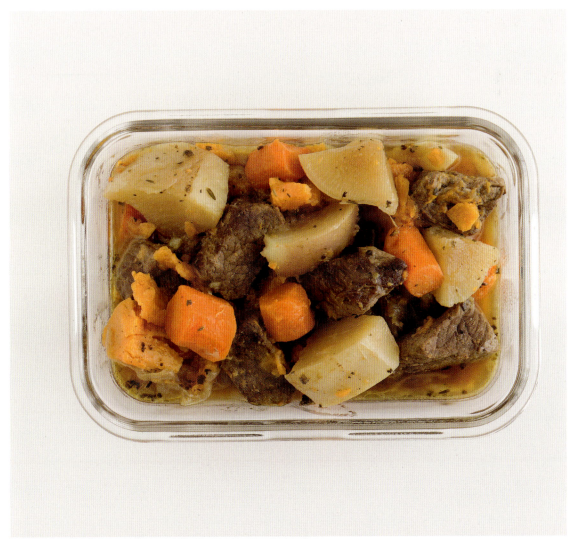

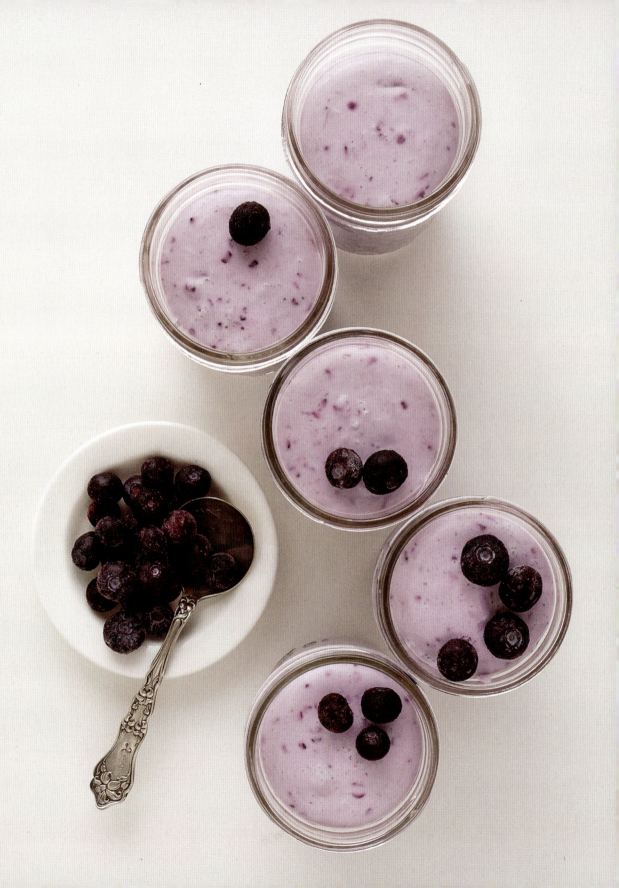

BLUEBERRY MOUSSE

Don't be fooled by blueberries' low-key appearance: When it comes to nutrition, they pack a serious punch! They're one of the healthiest types of fruit you can choose. These little berries promote healthy digestion, help fight cancer, and even alleviate inflammation. It would be a shame to pass them up, especially when you get to enjoy them in this simple, refreshing dessert.

Prep time:
10 minutes
Cook time:
N/A
Yield:
5 servings

1 (14-ounce [392 ml]) can + 1 cup (240 ml) full-fat coconut milk

2 cups (300 g) frozen blueberries

2 tablespoons (30 ml) maple syrup

3 tablespoons (45 ml) warm water

1½ tablespoons (12 g) gelatin powder

1. Add the coconut milk, blueberries, and maple syrup to a food processor equipped with an S-blade. Blend until smooth, about 20 seconds.

2. In a small cup, combine the warm water and gelatin powder. Mix well until you obtain a smooth, gel-like paste. Add to the food processor and continue to blend for another 10 seconds.

3. Divide the blueberry mousse evenly among 5 containers and refrigerate for at least 3 hours, or until firm.

   Note: Store for up to 5 days in an airtight container in the refrigerator. Not suitable for freezing.

CHICKEN FRIED RICE SKILLET

Now that I follow an AIP-compliant diet, one of the things I miss most is Chinese takeout—especially chicken fried rice—for both its great taste and its convenience. But the good news is, you can re-create your old takeout favorite with AIP-compliant ingredients, and it tastes terrific! This skillet recipe delivers all the flavors and textures you've come to love in a good fried rice recipe, including the savory, spicy sauce, and best of all, it takes only half an hour to make!

Prep time:
15 minutes
Cook time:
15 minutes
Yield:
4 servings

1 pound (454 g) boneless skinless chicken breasts

1 pound (454 g) cauliflower florets

¾ pound (340 g) carrots

1 yellow onion (½ pound [227 g])

4 scallions

½ cup (120 ml) coconut aminos, divided

2 tablespoons (30 ml) extra-virgin olive oil, divided

1¾ teaspoons sea salt, divided

1 teaspoon garlic powder, divided

1 teaspoon ginger powder, divided

1. Dice the chicken breasts into ⅓-inch (8 mm) pieces. Rice the cauliflower florets (see directions on page 177). Peel and dice the carrots into ¼-inch (6 mm) pieces. Mince the onion. Slice the scallions.

2. Heat 2 tablespoons (30 ml) of the coconut aminos and 1 tablespoon (15 ml) of the olive oil in a large skillet over medium-high heat. When hot, add the chicken and season with ¾ teaspoon of the salt. Mix well and cook, covered, until no longer pink, about 5 minutes. Use a slotted spatula to transfer to a large mixing bowl and return the skillet to the heat.

3. Heat 2 tablespoons (30 ml) of the coconut aminos in the skillet. When hot, add the carrots, onion, ½ teaspoon of the salt, ½ teaspoon of the garlic powder, and ½ teaspoon of the ginger powder. Mix well and cook, covered, until crisp-tender, about 5 minutes. Use a slotted spoon to transfer to the large mixing bowl with the chicken and return the skillet to the heat.

4. Heat the remaining 4 tablespoons (60 ml) coconut aminos and 1 tablespoon (15 ml) olive oil in the skillet. When hot, add the cauliflower rice, remaining ½ teaspoon salt, remaining ½ teaspoon garlic powder, and remaining ½ teaspoon ginger powder. Mix well and cook, covered, until crisp-tender, about 5 minutes.

5. When done, transfer the cauliflower rice to the large mixing bowl. Add the scallions and mix well. Check the seasoning and adjust to taste.

To assemble: Divide the Chicken Fried Rice Skillet evenly among 4 containers.

Note: Store for up to 5 days in an airtight container in the refrigerator, or freeze for up to 4 months.

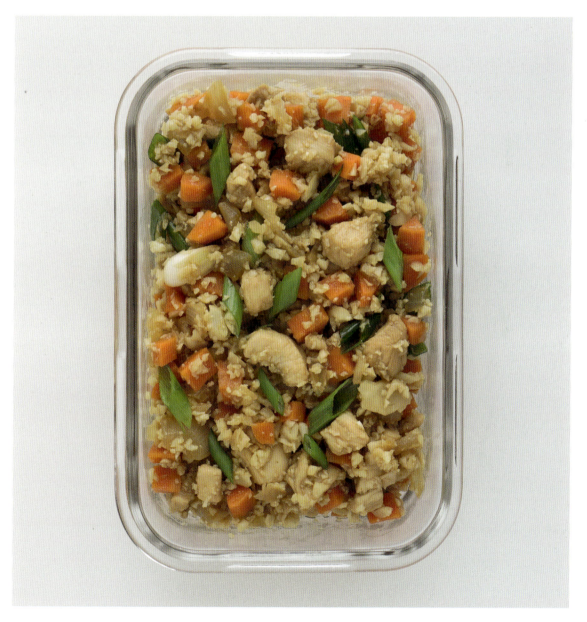

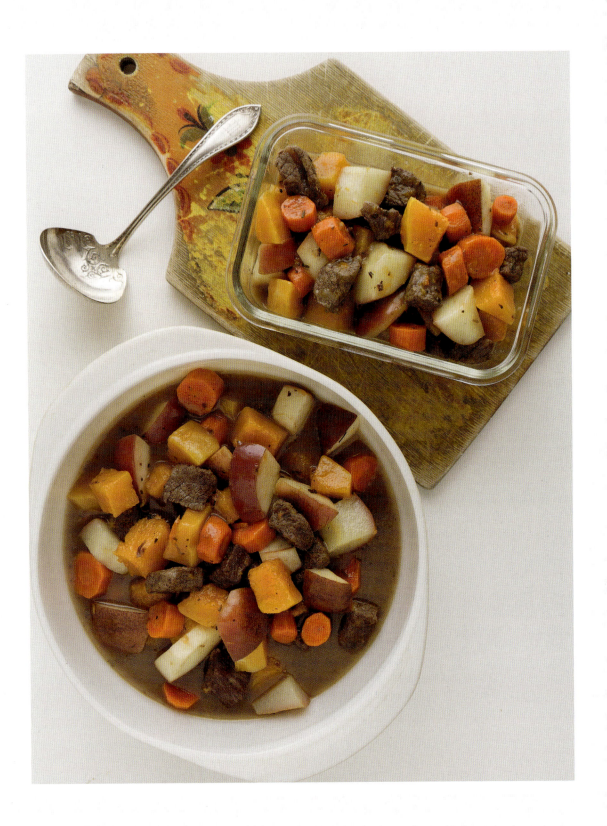

Chapter 13

HOLIDAYS MEAL PLAN

If you think that following a healing, AIP-compliant diet over the holidays is boring or tedious, you're about to be proved wrong! My Holidays Meal Plan is all about enjoying the season with wholesome, festive, creative dishes that'll also keep you on track healthwise.

And if you're considering throwing a big party for your family and friends, I've got your menu all lined up: The dishes in this meal plan also make up a single holiday meal for a big group. Just use the **Apple and Plum Breakfast Cake** for dessert, served with scoops of coconut-milk vanilla ice cream.

First on the menu is a **Beef, Pear, and Butternut Squash Stew**. This wonderfully fragrant stew is full of autumnal flavor, featuring winter squash, carrots, and—yes!—pears. And your snack is just as colorful: My sweet and sour **Pomegranate Gummies** are easy to make, are fun to eat, and deliver a daily dose of gut-healing gelatin. If you have extra time on your hands, you can turn these gummies into all sorts of fancy shapes using soft silicone molds. (Flowers and robots are my favorites!)

What about the main course? **Rosemary-Apple Roast Chicken with Delicata Squash, Cranberry Sauce, and Sweet Potato Mash** makes for a merry meal! In this recipe you'll also learn the technique of spatchcocking your chicken—a funny name for a technique that works wonders!—for a perfect, all-over golden crust and tender meat.

To wrap things up, we have a **Brussels Sprout Salad**, complete with pomegranate seeds and leftover chicken from the roast. It's ideal as a quick lunchtime salad on the go or as a side dish for your holiday party.

Kitchen note: Make sure you have 1 quart (1 L) of chicken or beef Bone Broth on hand for your batch-cooking session.

	BREAKFAST	LUNCH	DINNER	SNACK
DAY 1	Apple and Plum Breakfast Cake	Brussels Sprout Salad	Rosemary-Apple Roast Chicken	Pomegranate Gummies
DAY 2	Apple and Plum Breakfast Cake	Beef, Pear, and Butternut Squash Stew	Brussels Sprout Salad	Pomegranate Gummies
DAY 3	Apple and Plum Breakfast Cake	Brussels Sprout Salad	Rosemary-Apple Roast Chicken	Pomegranate Gummies
DAY 4	Apple and Plum Breakfast Cake	Beef, Pear, and Butternut Squash Stew	Brussels Sprout Salad	Pomegranate Gummies
DAY 5	Apple and Plum Breakfast Cake	Rosemary-Apple Roast Chicken	Beef, Pear, and Butternut Squash Stew	Pomegranate Gummies

EXTRA SERVINGS: 1 Beef, Pear, and Butternut Squash Stew +
1 Apple and Plum Breakfast Cake + 1 Rosemary-Apple Roast Chicken

Shopping List

PRODUCE

1 orange

1 pomegranate

2 celery ribs

3 red apples

3 firm red pears

1 cup + 2 tablespoons (240 ml + 30 ml) freshly
    squeezed lemon juice

1⅓ cups (315 ml) orange juice

3 cups (720 ml) pomegranate juice

5 ounces (140 g) pitted prunes

4 carrots (½ pound [227 g])

¾ pound (340 g) fresh cranberries

1 pound (454 g) Brussels sprouts

1 delicata squash (1½ pounds [680 g])

2 pounds (908 g) sweet potatoes

1 butternut squash (2¾ pounds [1250 g])

MEAT/SEAFOOD

1½ cups (210 g) diced cooked chicken

½ pound (227 g) bacon

1½ pounds (680 g) beef stew meat

1 chicken (4 pounds [1818 g])

1 quart (1 L) beef or chicken Bone Broth
    (page 180)

HERBS AND SPICES

1 bay leaf

½ teaspoon ginger powder

1 teaspoon garlic powder

1½ teaspoons ground cinnamon

1½ tablespoons (3 g) minced fresh rosemary

1½ tablespoons (3 g) dried sage

PANTRY ITEMS

½ teaspoon baking powder

5 tablespoons + 1 teaspoon (100 g + 7 g) honey

5½ tablespoons (44 g) gelatin powder

¼ cup + 2 tablespoons (60 ml + 30 ml) maple
    syrup

⅔ cup (80 g) arrowroot flour

1 cup (120 g) coconut flour

1 cup (235 ml) full-fat coconut milk

1 (15-ounce [420 g]) can pumpkin puree

OTHER

Coconut oil

Extra-virgin olive oil

Sea salt

Equipment and Tools

15 containers for your meals + 5 containers for
    snacks (see pages 32 to 33)

baking dish (9 x 5 inches [23 x 12.5 cm])

baking dish (11 x 7 inches [28 x 18 cm])

broiler pan or large rimmed baking sheet
    (12 x 17 inches [30.5 x 43 cm])

chef's knife

cutting board

food processor with slicing blade

measuring cups and spoons

mixing bowls

potato masher

pots and pans

rubber spatula

slotted spatula

stockpot

vegetable peeler

whisk

wooden spoon

Batch-Cooking Directions

1. Reminder: *The morning before*, defrost the meat/fish if frozen. Make sure you have 1 quart (1 L) of chicken or beef **Bone Broth** (page 180) on hand. Prepare your containers.

2. Start your batch-cooking session with the **Beef, Pear, and Butternut Squash Stew** (page 167). Complete steps 1 through 3. Set a timer for 1 hour.

3. While the stew meat is cooking, prep the vegetables for the stew as described in step 4. Also make the **Pomegranate Gummies** (page 169), steps 1 through 4, and refrigerate.

4. Prep the sweet potatoes for the **Sweet Potato Mash** (page 184), step 1, and start cooking, following step 2. Set a timer for 20 minutes.

5. When the timer for the stew goes off, add the butternut squash and carrots to the stockpot (step 5, page 167). Set a timer for 50 minutes.

6. When the sweet potatoes are done, complete step 3 of the **Sweet Potato Mash** (page 184) and set aside.

7. Preheat the oven to 350°F (180°C or gas mark 4) and place the rack in the middle. Complete the **Apple and Plum Breakfast Cake** (page 170), steps 1 through 5, and bake as described in step 6. Set a timer for 35 minutes.

8. When the timer goes off for the stew, add the pears and continue to cook for an additional 10 minutes. When done, allow the stew to cool slightly and assemble.

9. Remove the **Apple and Plum Breakfast Cake** (page 170) from the oven and let cool completely before cutting and storing. Increase the oven's heat to 400°F (200°C or gas mark 6).

10. Complete the **Rosemary-Apple Roast Chicken with Delicata Squash, Cranberry Sauce, and Sweet Potato Mash** (page 173), steps 1 through 4. Set a timer for 60 minutes.

11. Complete the **Brussels Sprout Salad** (page 174), steps 1 through 4. You will have to wait for the roast chicken to be done to add some cooked chicken to this salad and assemble. Also make the **Vinaigrette** (page 185).

12. When the roast chicken is done, complete step 5 (page 173) and assemble.

13. Don't forget to cut the gummies when the gelatin is firm.

BEEF, PEAR, *and* BUTTERNUT SQUASH STEW

A good beef stew recipe is a lot like a little black dress: a reliable must-have that you'll use again and again. If you don't already have a great beef stew recipe in your "wardrobe," you'll thank me for this one! Like any other stew prepared on the stovetop, it needs to simmer for over two hours for the meat to reach that perfectly tender stage, but other than that, there's very little prep involved.

Prep time:
12 minutes

Cook time:
2 hours 10 minutes

Yield:
4 servings

1½ pounds (680 g) beef stew meat

⅓ cup (40 g) arrowroot flour

1 teaspoon garlic powder

1 teaspoon sea salt

¼ cup (60 ml) olive oil

1 quart (1 L) beef or chicken Bone Broth (page 180)

1 bay leaf

1½ tablespoons (3 g) dried sage

1 butternut squash (2¾ pounds [1250 g])

4 carrots (½ pound [227 g])

3 firm red pears

1. Add the meat, arrowroot flour, garlic powder, and salt to a resealable plastic bag. Close the bag and shake to coat.

2. Heat the olive oil in a stockpot over medium heat. When hot, add the meat and brown on all sides. You may have to do this in two batches.

3. Add the broth, bay leaf, and sage. Cover, bring to a boil over high heat, then decrease the heat to medium-low and simmer for 1 hour.

4. Meanwhile, cut off the top and bottom of the butternut squash and discard. Peel and slice in half lengthwise. Scoop out and discard the seeds, then chop into 1-inch (2.5 cm) pieces. Peel and slice the carrots. Core and chop the pears.

5. Add the butternut squash and carrots to the stockpot, and continue to cook for 50 minutes.

6. Add the pears and cook for an additional 10 minutes. When done, discard the bay leaf, check the seasoning, and adjust the salt to taste.

To assemble: Divide the stew evenly among 4 glass containers.

Note: Store for up to 5 days in an airtight container in the refrigerator, or freeze for up to 4 months.

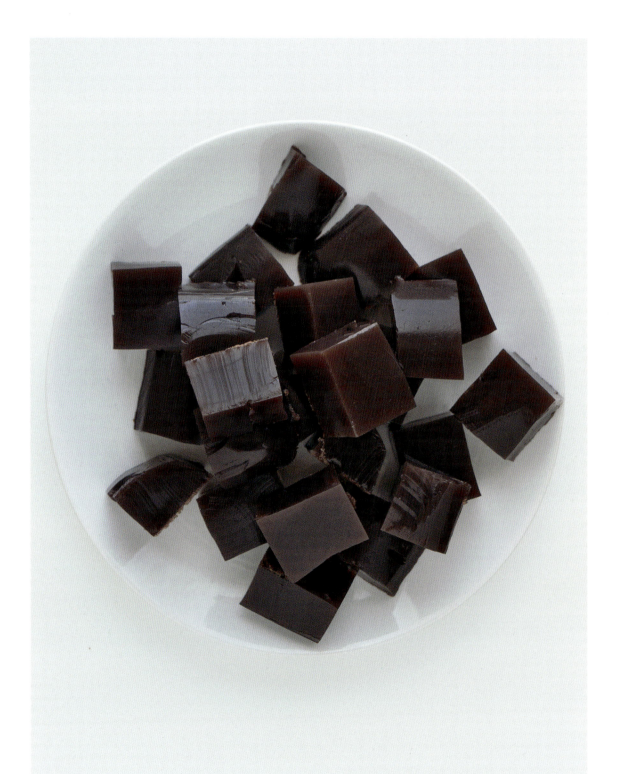

POMEGRANATE GUMMIES

These bright-red gummies are such fun to make, especially if you pour the prepared gelatin into soft silicone molds to make interesting shapes. Get the kids involved: They'll love to unmold the gummies with their little fingers! These treats might look like candy, but they're sweetened only with honey, and they come with a healthy dose of hidden protein in the form of gelatin powder. It's a potent gut-healing agent and is also excellent for hair, skin, and nails.

Prep time:
5 minutes
Cook time:
5 minutes
Yield:
5 servings

3 cups (720 ml) pomegranate juice

4 tablespoons (32 g) gelatin powder

2 tablespoons (40 g) honey, or more to taste

1. Lightly grease the bottom of a 9 x 5-inch (23 x 12.5 cm) glass baking dish.

2. Add the pomegranate juice to a saucepan and sprinkle the gelatin powder over the juice. Don't add the gelatin all at once or it will clump. Instead, add it in stages and wait for it to melt before adding more.

3. When the gelatin is completely melted, add the honey and heat the mixture gently over medium heat, stirring regularly, for 2 to 3 minutes.

4. Pour the liquid into the prepared baking dish and refrigerate until the gelatin is firm, at least 4 hours.

5. Cut into 2-inch (5 cm) squares for easy portioning before storing.

   To assemble: Divide the gummies evenly among 5 glass containers.

   Note: Store for up to 7 days in an airtight container in the refrigerator. Not suitable for freezing.

APPLE and PLUM BREAKFAST CAKE

This festive breakfast cake makes for a welcome departure from the usual dinner-for-breakfast routine. And it's adaptable, too: As you work your way through the reintroduction process (see page 13), try adding some nuts, such as walnuts or pecans, to the batter. Pro tip: Make your own AIP-friendly baking powder by mixing 2 tablespoons (16 g) cream of tartar with 1 tablespoon (8 g) baking soda.

Prep time:
20 minutes
Cook time:
35 minutes
Yield:
6 servings

Coconut oil for greasing the baking dish

1 cup (120 g) coconut flour

⅓ cup (40 g) arrowroot flour

½ teaspoon baking powder

⅛ teaspoon sea salt

2 red apples

5 ounces (140 g) pitted prunes

1 (15-ounce [420 g]) can pumpkin puree

½ cup (120 ml) coconut milk

6 tablespoons (90 ml) maple syrup

1½ teaspoons ground cinnamon

½ teaspoon ginger powder

1½ tablespoons (12 g) gelatin powder

¼ cup (60 ml) warm water

1. Preheat the oven to 350°F (180°C or gas mark 4) and place the rack in the middle. Grease an 11 x 7-inch (28 x 18 cm) baking dish with coconut oil.

2. In a small mixing bowl, combine the coconut flour, arrowroot flour, baking powder, and salt. Set aside. Peel, core, and dice the apples. Chop the prunes.

3. In a large mixing bowl, combine the pumpkin puree, coconut milk, maple syrup, cinnamon, ginger, apples, and prunes. Mix well with a rubber spatula.

4. Add the gelatin powder and warm water to a cup. Stir well, making sure the powder is completely dissolved, then incorporate the gelatin mixture into the pumpkin batter.

5. Add the dry ingredients to the pumpkin batter and mix well with a rubber spatula or your hands.

6. Transfer the batter to the prepared baking dish and bake in the oven for 35 minutes, until the edges turn golden brown and a toothpick inserted close to the center comes out dry.

7. Allow to cool completely before slicing.

   To assemble: Divide the cake slices evenly among 6 glass containers.

   Note: Store for up to 5 days in an airtight container in the refrigerator, or freeze for up to 4 months.

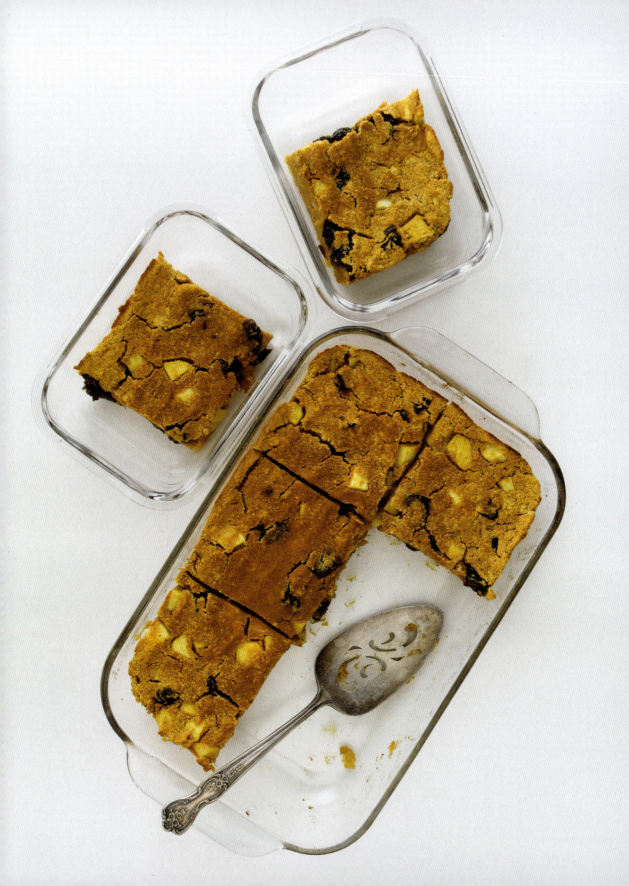

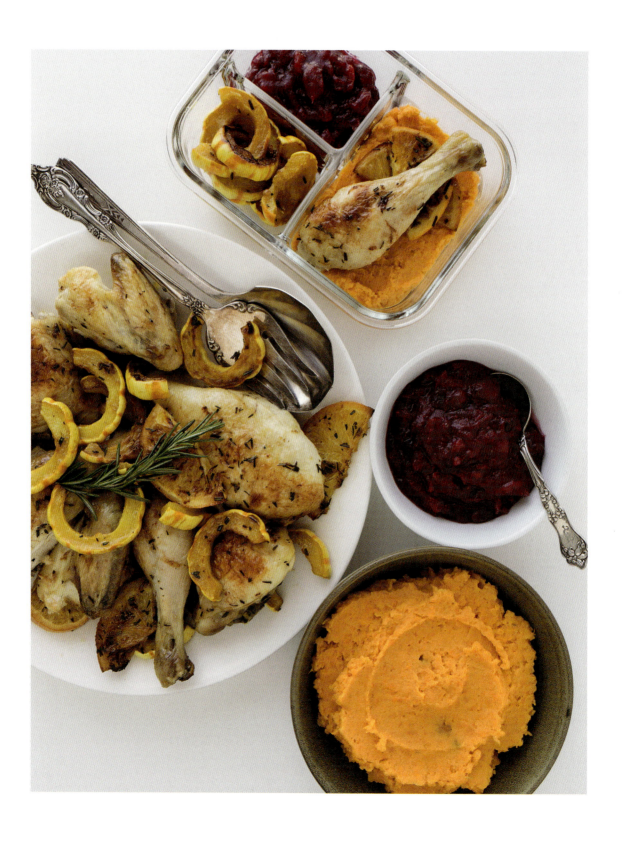

ROSEMARY-APPLE ROAST CHICKEN *with* DELICATA SQUASH, CRANBERRY SAUCE, *and* SWEET POTATO MASH

Ever spatchcocked a chicken before? With this technique, the chicken cooks faster and more evenly. Here's how to do it: Place the chicken breast-side down on a cutting board. Using kitchen shears or a chef's knife, cut along both sides of the backbone. (Use the backbone to make chicken Bone Broth, page 180!) Flip the chicken over and press down firmly on the breastbone with your hands to flatten. That's it! Use leftover chicken to make the Brussels Sprout Salad (page 174).

Prep time:
20 minutes
Cook time:
60 minutes
Yield:
4 servings

1 chicken (4 pounds [1818 g])

2 tablespoons (30 ml) olive oil, divided, plus extra for greasing the pan

2 teaspoons sea salt, divided

1½ tablespoons (3 g) minced fresh rosemary, divided

1 delicata squash (1½ pounds [680 g])

1 orange, sliced (with peel)

FOR THE CRANBERRY SAUCE:

¾ pound (340 g) fresh cranberries

1 cup (240 ml) orange juice

3 tablespoons (60 g) honey, or more to taste

1 recipe prepared Sweet Potato Mash (page 184)

1. Preheat the oven to 400°F (200°C or gas mark 6) and place the rack in the middle. Line a rimmed pan with aluminum foil and grease the bottom.

2. Spatchcock the chicken following the instructions above, then place in the center of the broiler pan, skin-side up. Rub with 1 tablespoon (15 ml) of the olive oil and season with 1 teaspoon of the salt and 1 tablespoon (2 g) of the rosemary.

3. Cut off the top and bottom of the squash and discard, then cut in half lengthwise. Scoop out and discard the seeds. Slice the squash into ¼-inch (6 mm) pieces and transfer to a mixing bowl. Add the sliced orange, remaining 1 tablespoon (15 ml) olive oil, remaining 1 teaspoon salt, and remaining ½ tablespoon (1 g) rosemary. Mix well and arrange on the pan around the chicken. Cook in the oven, basting halfway through, until the chicken is nicely browned and the thick part of the thighs reaches an internal temperature of 165°F (74°C), about 60 minutes.

4. Meanwhile, make the cranberry sauce. Add the cranberries and orange juice to a saucepan. Cook over medium heat until the cranberries start to pop, about 10 minutes. Sweeten with honey.

5. When the chicken is done, transfer to a cutting board and let rest for 10 minutes before cutting.

To assemble: Divide the chicken, squash, sweet potato mash, and cranberry sauce evenly among 4 glass containers.

Note: Store for up to 5 days in an airtight container in the refrigerator, or freeze for up to 4 months.

BRUSSELS SPROUT SALAD

This hearty Brussels sprout salad is really versatile. You can serve it as a side dish during a holiday meal or as a stand-alone salad for a quick lunch at home or at work. Pro tip: Take a shortcut on the prep time and get prepackaged shaved Brussels sprouts from the grocery store!

Prep time:
15 minutes
Cook time:
10 minutes
Yield:
4 servings

½ pound (227 g) bacon

1 red apple

½ cup (120 ml) lemon juice

1 pound (454 g) Brussels sprouts

2 celery ribs

1 pomegranate

1½ cups (210 g) diced cooked chicken

1 recipe Vinaigrette (page 185)

1. Cut the bacon into 1-inch (2.5 cm) pieces. Add to a skillet and cook over medium heat until golden, about 10 minutes, stirring occasionally. When done, transfer to a paper towel–lined plate with a slotted spatula.

2. Meanwhile, quarter and core the apple, and thinly slice. Transfer to a bowl and cover with the lemon juice to soak while you prepare the rest of the ingredients. (This will slow the oxidation process and prevent browning.)

3. Trim and discard the stems from the Brussels sprouts. Slice using a food processor equipped with a slicing blade. Transfer to a large mixing bowl.

4. Thinly slice the celery, seed the pomegranate, and drain the apples. Add these to the Brussels sprouts, along with the bacon and chicken. Mix well.

To assemble: Divide the salad evenly among 4 glass jar containers. I recommend keeping the dressing on the side, adding it right before serving.

Note: Store for up to 5 days in an airtight container in the refrigerator. Not suitable for freezing.

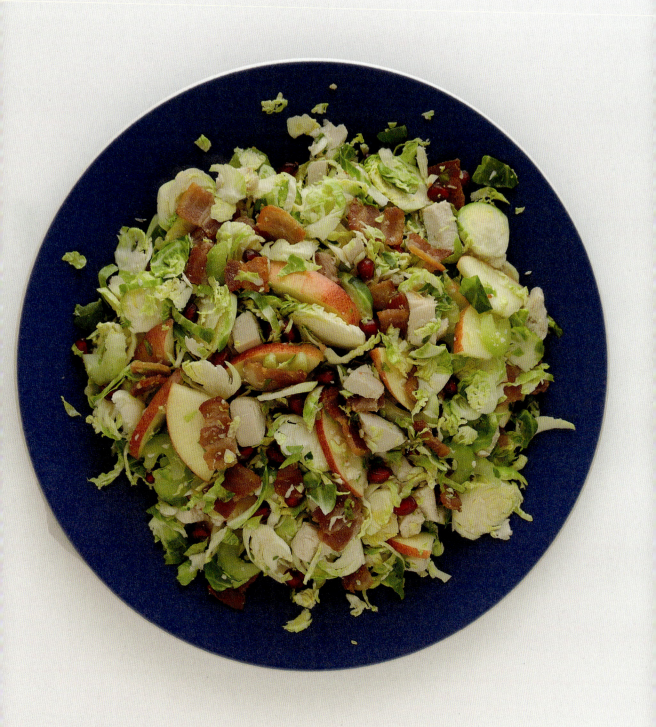

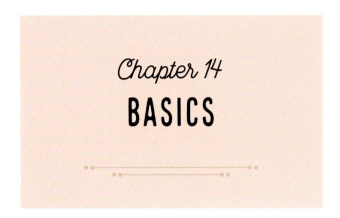

Chapter 14
BASICS

BUTTERNUT SQUASH RICE

This creative butternut squash recipe provides a convenient alternative to rice during the elimination stage. Use this colorful, high-fiber butternut squash rice as a side dish to accompany meat, poultry, and seafood. Make sure you give the Turmeric Squash Risotto (page 87) or the Moroccan Chicken (page 128) a try!

Prep time:
10 minutes
Cook time:
5 minutes
Yield:
4 or 5 servings

1 butternut squash (2 pounds [908 g])

2 tablespoons (30 ml) coconut oil

Sea salt to taste

1. Cut off the top and bottom of the butternut squash and discard. Peel and slice in half lengthwise. Scoop out and discard the seeds, then chop the flesh into 1-inch (2.5 cm) pieces.

2. Transfer to a food processor equipped with an S-blade and chop/pulse until the butternut squash pieces turn into small grains, about 10 seconds. (Don't overprocess the squash or it will turn to paste.) You may have to do this in several batches.

3. Heat the coconut oil in a large skillet over medium heat. When hot, add the butternut squash rice, cover, and cook, stirring occasionally, until crisp-tender, about 5 minutes. (Don't overcook the squash or it will get mushy!) Season with salt to taste.

Note: Store for up to 5 days in an airtight container in the refrigerator, or freeze for up to 4 months.

CAULIFLOWER RICE

Eating healthy is all about making better food choices and finding ways to make "eating right" easy and enjoyable. That way, your new eating plan becomes a new way of life rather than a quick-fix diet. That's why I love to use smart swaps in my AIP kitchen, replacing traditional basics (such as rice, mashed potatoes, or pasta) with healthier options. Cauliflower rice is a great example. It looks very much like normal rice, and it can act as a nourishing side dish or a versatile base ingredient for more elaborate meals like the Cuban Mojo Chicken (page 41), Thai Curry Meatballs (page 132), or Chicken Fried Rice Skillet (page 160).

Prep time:
10 minutes
Cook time:
10 minutes
Yield:
6 servings

1 head cauliflower (2 pounds [908 g])

2 tablespoons (30 ml) coconut oil, olive oil, or avocado oil

Sea salt to taste

1. Discard all the green leaves, then core and chop the cauliflower into small florets.

2. Transfer the florets to a food processor equipped with an S-blade and chop/pulse until the florets become small grains, about 10 seconds. (Don't overprocess the florets or they will turn to paste.) You may have to do this in several batches.

3. Heat the coconut oil in a large skillet over medium heat. When hot, add the cauliflower rice and cook uncovered, stirring frequently, for 8 to 10 minutes, or until tender. Don't let the cauliflower rice get mushy! Season with salt to taste.

   Note: Store for up to 5 days in an airtight container in the refrigerator, or freeze for up to 4 months.

ASIAN DRESSING

Citrus and freshly grated ginger combine to make this uplifting, savory Asian dressing incredibly flavorful. (Do freshly grate your ginger—a small handheld grater makes the job a breeze.) Feel free to use additional ginger for an extra kick!

Prep time:
5 minutes
Cook time:
N/A
Yield:
1 cup (240 ml)

½ cup (120 ml) extra-virgin olive oil

⅓ cup (80 ml) freshly squeezed orange juice

2 tablespoons (30 ml) coconut aminos

½ tablespoon (10 g) honey

Juice of ½ lime

1 teaspoon grated fresh ginger

Pinch sea salt

1. Combine all the ingredients in a glass jar with a tight-fitting lid and shake well.

2. Keep refrigerated until needed. Remove from the refrigerator 10 minutes before serving to allow the olive oil to soften. Shake well again before using.

Note: Store for up to 7 days in an airtight container in the refrigerator.

BASIL-CILANTRO PESTO

The antioxidant benefits of fresh basil, paired with the detoxing properties of fresh cilantro, make this condiment a potent healing elixir! Add it to your vegetables and meat for a bright, fresh boost of flavor. Pro tip: When cooking with pesto, add it during the last 5 minutes of cooking to maximize flavor and nutrients.

Prep time:
5 minutes
Cook time:
N/A
Yield:
1 cup (240 g)

3 ounces (84 g) fresh basil (about 1 large bunch)

3 ounces (84 g) fresh cilantro

4 cloves garlic (omit for low-FODMAP)

½ cup (120 ml) olive oil, or more to taste

1½ teaspoons lemon juice

Sea salt to taste

1. Cut off and discard the hard stems of the fresh herbs (if any), then roughly chop. Mince the garlic.

2. Add all the ingredients to a high-speed blender or a food processor equipped with an S-blade. Blend for 30 seconds or until the pesto reaches the desired consistency. Adjust the quantity of olive oil and salt to taste.

3. Transfer to an airtight container and refrigerate until needed.

Note: Store for up to 7 days in an airtight container in the refrigerator.

BAKED SPAGHETTI SQUASH

For a nutritious, filling side dish, swap traditional pasta for spaghetti squash noodles. Spaghetti squash is an excellent source of fiber and is fairly inexpensive, which makes it a great addition to your AIP kitchen.

Prep time:
5 minutes
Cook time:
30 minutes oven
10 minutes pressure cooker
Yield: 4 servings

1 spaghetti squash, about 3 pounds (1362 g)

OVEN DIRECTIONS

1. Preheat the oven to 400°F (200°C or gas mark 6) and place the rack in the middle.

2. Cut off the top and bottom of the spaghetti squash with a serrated knife and discard. Slice it in half lengthwise. Scoop out the seeds and discard. Place both halves, cut-side down, in a baking dish and add 1 inch (2.5 cm) of water. Bake in the oven for 30 minutes, until the skins soften and give a little when you press them with your finger.

3. Transfer the spaghetti squash to a plate and allow to cool slightly before scraping out the flesh with a fork, making spaghetti noodles.

ELECTRIC PRESSURE COOKER DIRECTIONS

1. Add 1 cup (240 ml) of water to the stainless steel container of your pressure cooker. Place the trivet inside.

2. Cut off the top and bottom of the spaghetti squash with a serrated knife and discard. Slice it in half lengthwise. Scoop out the seeds and discard. Place both halves on top of the trivet, cut sides facing each other.

3. Close the lid of the pressure cooker and make sure the pressure knob is in the SEALING position. Using the display panel, select MANUAL, high pressure, and adjust the cooking time to 10 minutes using the +/- buttons.

4. When the pressure cooker beeps and the cooking time is done, press CANCEL and quick-release the pressure by switching the pressure knob to the VENTING position.

5. Transfer the spaghetti squash to a plate and allow to cool slightly before scraping out the flesh with a fork, making spaghetti noodles.

BONE BROTH

A number of recipes in this book call for bone broth, either chicken or beef, so you should definitely have a batch or two on hand. Vary the "flavor" of your bone broth by using either chicken or beef bones. Also, adding a few chicken feet to the simmering broth will increase the collagen content, thus resulting in a more gelatinous broth (the broth will turn "jiggly" when refrigerated but will liquefy when reheated).

Prep time:
5 minutes
Cook time:
variable
Yield:
3 quarts (2.7 L)

2½ to 3 pounds (1135 to 1362 g) chicken or beef bones

3 quarts (2.7 L) water

1 tablespoon (15 ml) apple cider vinegar

SLOW COOKER DIRECTIONS

1. Place the bones at the bottom of a 6-quart (5.4 L) slow cooker, then cover with water (you may have to adjust the quantity of water to cover the bones entirely). Add the vinegar. Close the lid and simmer on low for 12 to 24 hours.

2. Discard the bones with a slotted spatula and strain the liquid to remove all the little bits and pieces. Allow the broth to cool before refrigerating or freezing.

PRESSURE COOKER DIRECTIONS

1. Place the bones in the Instant Pot and cover with water (no higher than the maximum line), then add the vinegar.

2. Close the lid, making sure the valve is in the SEALING position. Press MANUAL and adjust the cooking time to 120 minutes using the +/- buttons.

3. When the time is up, let the pressure release naturally. Discard the bones with a slotted spatula and strain the liquid to remove all the little bits and pieces. Allow the broth to cool completely before refrigerating or freezing.

Note: Store for up to 7 days in an airtight container in the refrigerator, or freeze for up to 4 months.

BROCCOLI MASH

Wondering how to "eat your broccoli," but bored with the steamed or roasted versions? Been there! That's exactly why I created this ultra-easy and oh-so-convenient broccoli mash recipe. Now you get to enjoy a comforting side dish that's also chock-full of health-promoting vegetables. Win-win!

Prep time:
5 minutes
Cook time:
15 minutes
Yield:
4 servings

1 pound (454 g) broccoli florets

1 white sweet potato (¾ pound [340 g]), peeled and chopped

½ cup (120 ml) full-fat coconut milk

Sea salt to taste

1. Place the broccoli and chopped sweet potato in a large saucepan and cover with water. Bring to a boil over high heat, then reduce the heat to medium and cook until tender, about 15 minutes.

2. Drain the water and transfer the vegetables to a food processor equipped with an S-blade. Add the coconut milk and process until creamy and smooth, about 30 seconds. You may have to do this in several batches. Season to taste with salt.

Note: Store for up to 5 days in an airtight container in the refrigerator, or freeze for up to 4 months.

MAYONNAISE

Use this AIP-friendly mayo as a dressing for all your salads or as a dip for freshly cut vegetables. Pro tip: This mayo tends to solidify when refrigerated, so you'll want to take it out of the fridge about 20 minutes before serving for a creamier consistency. Try adding garlic powder to taste for an AIP aioli!

Prep time:
5 minutes
Cook time:
N/A
Yield:
1 cup (235 g)

⅓ cup (80 ml) avocado oil

⅓ cup (80 ml) extra-virgin olive oil

⅓ cup (80 g) palm shortening

1 teaspoon lemon juice

Pinch sea salt

1. Combine all the ingredients in a mixing bowl and beat with a hand mixer for about 30 seconds until you obtain a smooth, creamy texture. Check the seasoning and adjust the salt to taste.

Note: Store for up to 7 days in an airtight container in the refrigerator. Not suitable for freezing.

DAIRY-FREE CHEESE SAUCE

This dairy-free, plant-based cheese sauce makes a creamy, savory topping for vegetables and proteins alike. But what gives this sauce its cheesy taste? Nutritional yeast! "Nooch" comes in the form of little golden flakes (or powder) and has a high protein content. Be sure to try this healthy cheese sauce in the Broccoli and Cheese Stuffed Sweet Potatoes (page 142)!

Prep time:
5 minutes
Cook time:
10 minutes
Yield:
2¼ cups (540 ml) or
1½ pounds (504 g)

1 pound (454 g) cauliflower florets

½ cup (35 g) nutritional yeast

⅓ cup (80 ml) chicken Bone Broth (page 180)

1 teaspoon sea salt

1. Add the cauliflower florets to a pot and cover with water. Bring to a boil over high heat, then reduce the heat to medium and cook until tender, about 10 minutes.

2. Drain the water and transfer the cauliflower to a high-speed blender. Add the nutritional yeast, chicken broth, and salt. Blend on high until smooth and creamy, about 30 seconds. Check the seasoning and adjust to taste.

3. Serve immediately or store in an airtight container in the refrigerator until needed.

   Note: Store for up to 7 days in an airtight container in the refrigerator, or freeze for up to 4 months.

MARINARA SAUCE

Have you been missing good spaghetti sauce since starting your AIP eating plan? If so, you'll love this thick, faux-tomato sauce, perfectly seasoned with Italian spices like basil, marjoram, and oregano. Try it in the Italian Meatballs (page 44) or the Zucchini Boats (page 73)!

Prep time:
10 minutes
Cook time:
30 minutes
Yield:
4 cups (960 ml) or
24 ounces (672 g)

½ pound (225 g) beets

½ pound (225 g) carrots

½ pound (225 g) sweet potatoes

1⅓ cups (320 ml) chicken Bone Broth (page 180)

3 tablespoons (45 ml) coconut aminos

2 tablespoons (30 ml) balsamic vinegar

2 teaspoons (2 g) dried basil

2 teaspoons (2 g) dried marjoram

1½ teaspoons dried oregano

1½ teaspoons salt

1 teaspoon garlic powder (omit for low-FODMAP)

1. Peel and dice the beets, carrots, and sweet potatoes. Add to a pot, cover with water, and bring to a boil over high heat. Reduce the heat to medium and cook, covered, until tender, about 30 minutes.

2. Drain the water when the root vegetables are done and transfer them to a food processor equipped with an S-blade. Add the chicken broth, coconut aminos, balsamic vinegar, herbs, salt, and garlic powder. Process on high until smooth, 30 to 45 seconds.

Note: Store for up to 5 days in an airtight container in the refrigerator, or freeze for up to 4 months.

NO-COOK BBQ SAUCE

This AIP-compliant BBQ sauce is big on rich, smoky taste: You'd never know that there's no added sugar or tomato in sight! Use it with slow-cooked ribs, for chicken wings, or to prepare my BBQ Party Meatballs (page 146).

Prep time:
5 minutes
Cook time:
N/A
Yield:
2 cups (480 ml)

1½ cups (370 g) unsweetened applesauce

¼ cup (60 ml) apple cider vinegar

¼ cup (60 ml) coconut aminos

2½ tablespoons (50 g) blackstrap molasses

1½ teaspoons garlic powder

½ teaspoon ginger powder

½ teaspoon onion powder

1. Combine all the ingredients in a bowl and stir well.

2. Transfer to a glass container with a lid. Refrigerate until needed.

   Note: Store for up to 7 days in an airtight container in the refrigerator, or freeze for up to 4 months.

SWEET POTATO MASH

Sweet potatoes won't spike your blood sugar the same way regular potatoes will: They're part of the family of slow-burning carbs, thanks to their high fiber content. Use them to make potato mash, oven-baked sweet potato wedges (page 111), soups (page 55), and skillets (page 77).

Prep time:
5 minutes
Cook time:
20 minutes
Yield:
4 servings

2 pounds (908 g) sweet potatoes

½ cup (120 ml) full-fat coconut milk

Sea salt to taste

Note: Use either orange or white sweet potatoes

1. Peel and dice the sweet potatoes into ½-inch (1 cm) pieces.

2. Place in a large saucepan, cover with water, and bring to a boil over high heat. Reduce the heat to medium and cook, partially covered, until fully tender, 15 to 20 minutes.

3. When the potatoes are done, drain the water, add the coconut milk, and mash with a potato masher. (You may adjust the quantity of coconut milk to make the mash more or less creamy.) Add salt to taste.

   Note: Store for up to 5 days in an airtight container in the refrigerator, or freeze for up to 4 months.

QUICK GRAVY

To make a gravy, you can either use any cooking juices or pan drippings you have on hand or start from scratch with a mix of chicken broth and coconut milk. Whatever liquid you use, make sure you have 1¼ cups (300 ml) to work with in total. The final color and taste will vary slightly, depending on the type of liquid base you are using.

Prep time:
5 minutes
Cook time:
5 minutes
Yield:
1¼ cups (300 ml)

1 tablespoon (8 g) arrowroot flour

¾ cup (180 ml) chicken Bone Broth (page 180), divided

½ cup (120 ml) full-fat coconut milk

1½ tablespoons (23 ml) coconut aminos

½ teaspoon onion powder

½ teaspoon sea salt

1. In a small cup, dissolve the arrowroot flour in ¼ cup (60 ml) of the chicken broth.

2. To a saucepan, add the remaining ½ cup (120 ml) chicken broth, coconut milk, coconut aminos, onion powder, and salt. Stir well and bring to a boil over medium-high heat.

3. When the liquid boils, turn off the heat and add the arrowroot mixture, stirring with a whisk until you obtain a smooth sauce, about 20 seconds. Check the seasoning and adjust to taste.

Note: Store for up to 5 days in an airtight container in the refrigerator, or freeze for up to 4 months.

VINAIGRETTE

This simple, citrusy vinaigrette will liven up your salads all year long!

Prep time:
5 minutes
Cook time: N/A
Yield:
1 cup (240 ml)

½ cup (120 ml) extra-virgin olive oil

⅓ cup (80 ml) freshly squeezed orange juice

2 tablespoons (30 ml) lemon juice

1 teaspoon honey

Pinch sea salt

1. Combine all the ingredients in a glass jar with a tight-fitting lid and shake well.

2. Keep refrigerated until needed. Remove from the refrigerator 10 minutes before serving to allow the olive oil to soften. Shake well again before using.

Note: Store for up to 7 days in an airtight container in the refrigerator. Not suitable for freezing.

TERIYAKI SAUCE

This wheat-free teriyaki sauce makes a terrific addition to your AIP kitchen! Use it in your vegetable stir-fries or as a base for flavorful meals like the Teriyaki Pineapple Chicken (page 113) or the Teriyaki Chicken Wings (page 141).

Prep time:
5 minutes
Cook time:
5 minutes
Yield:
¾ cup (180 ml)

¾ cup (180 ml) coconut aminos

2 tablespoons (30 ml) maple syrup

1 teaspoon garlic powder

1 teaspoon ginger powder

½ teaspoon onion powder

½ teaspoon sea salt

1 tablespoon (8 g) arrowroot flour

1. Combine all the ingredients except the arrowroot starch in a saucepan. Bring to a low boil over medium heat, stirring constantly.

2. When the liquid boils, turn off the heat, sprinkle in the arrowroot starch, and whisk until the flour is completely dissolved and the liquid thickens, about 20 seconds.

3. Transfer to a glass container with a lid. Refrigerate until needed.

   Note: Store for up to 5 days in an airtight container in the refrigerator, or freeze for up to 4 months.

TZATZIKI DRESSING

This Greek-inspired dairy-free dressing is light and so refreshing! Use it to prepare the Greek Salad (page 74) or any time you need a creamy condiment for your vegetables and proteins (especially chicken or lamb). Pro tip: Mince and freeze fresh herbs for convenient use later.

Prep time:
10 minutes
Cook time: **N/A**
Yield: **1½ cups (360 ml) or ¾ pound (340 g)**

1 English cucumber (¾ pound [340 g])

5 ounces (140 g) coconut yogurt

2 tablespoons (8 g) minced fresh dill

2 tablespoons (8 g) minced fresh mint

2 teaspoons (10 ml) freshly squeezed lemon juice

½ teaspoon sea salt

1. Peel the cucumber, scoop out and discard the seeds using a spoon, then chop.

2. Add all the ingredients to a food processor equipped with an S-blade and blend until smooth, about 15 seconds. Check the seasoning and adjust to taste. Transfer to a glass container and refrigerate until needed.

   Note: Store for up to 5 days in an airtight container in the refrigerator. Not suitable for freezing.

Additional Resources

Hey, let's be friends and stay connected!

Visit my blog, *A Squirrel in the Kitchen*, for AIP recipes and lifestyle tips for the Autoimmune Protocol. www.asquirrelinthekitchen.com

Subscribe to my newsletter to stay in the loop.

Join my Facebook group (www.facebook.com/groups/asquirrelinthekitchen) for daily discussions, cooking demos, live Q&As, and much more!

Get my other AIP cookbooks, *Simple French Paleo* and *The Autoimmune Protocol Made Simple*.

OTHER AUTOIMMUNE BLOGS
The Paleo Mom, www.thepaleomom.com
Autoimmune Wellness, www.autoimmunewellness.com
Phoenix Helix, www.phoenixhelix.com

FURTHER READING
The Paleo Approach by Sarah Ballantyne, Ph.D.
The Autoimmune Wellness Handbook by Mickey Trescott, NTP, and Angie Alt, NTC, CHC
A Simple Guide to the Paleo Autoimmune Protocol by Eileen Laird
The Autoimmune Solution by Amy Myers, M.D.
The Autoimmune Fix by Tom O'Bryan, DC, CCN, DACBN
The Wahls Protocol by Terry Wahls, M.D.
Hashimoto's Protocol by Izabella Wentz, Pharm.D., FASCP

MORE AUTOIMMUNE PROTOCOL COOKBOOKS
The Paleo Approach Cookbook by Sarah Ballantyne, Ph.D.
The Autoimmune Paleo Cookbook by Mickey Trescott, NTP
The Alternative Autoimmune Cookbook by Angie Alt
The Healing Kitchen by Alaena Haber, MS, OTR/L, and Sarah Ballantyne, Ph.D.
The Nutrient-Dense Kitchen by Mickey Trescott, NTP
He Won't Know It's Paleo by Breanna Emmitt
Nourish by Rachael Bryant

Acknowledgments

Behind every cookbook is a whole team of people supporting the author and recipe creator. Without all of you, this cookbook wouldn't have come to life the way it did, and I am forever grateful for your support and encouragement.

I want to take the time to acknowledge some of you.

Dr. Sarah Ballantyne, I am grateful for your dedication to the autoimmune community, your tireless work to create educational resources that help people regain their health, your guidance, and for, once again, writing the foreword for my cookbook.

Jill Alexander and the entire team at Fair Winds Press, thank you for your trust in me, your guidance, and your expertise in helping me publish a new AIP cookbook to help autoimmune warriors achieve their health goals.

My readers, followers, and all the autoimmune warriors, thanks for the fearless courage you demonstrate every day in taking your health into your own hands and becoming an active participant in your healing journey. Your example stands as a powerful motivation that keeps me moving forward on my own personal and professional journey!

Diane, Caroline, Rosalie, Lyse Marie, Joanna, Valerie, Lisa, Alice: You are all part of the Squirrel gang! Thank you for always showing up for me—you are the stars in my sky.

Kris, thank you for your steady and nurturing presence in my life and your undeniable talent as a recipe tester! I bless the day our paths crossed.

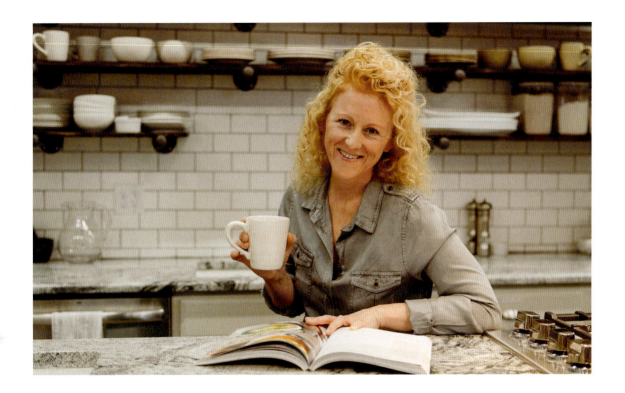

About the Author

Sophie Van Tiggelen is a passionate foodie, recipe developer, author, and photographer. Diagnosed with Hashimoto's thyroiditis in 2009, she used the Autoimmune Protocol (AIP) to reverse her condition and, today, Sophie lives a full and vibrant life free from the anxiety and flare-ups that often accompany autoimmune diseases.

With her food and lifestyle blog *A Squirrel in the Kitchen*, Sophie shares her AIP experience and empowers others to develop new habits to promote good health and wellness. Through years of experience, she has developed simple strategies to be successful on AIP, including numerous mouth-watering, allergen-free recipes that everyone (even those without autoimmune diseases) can enjoy.

Sophie is on a mission to make the Autoimmune Protocol—and all that it encompasses—more accessible and sustainable for anyone looking for a more nutritious, more delicious, more health-conscious life.

Index